# RAISING A BUNDLE OF JOY

A First Time Mom's Guide to That First Year

Elane Holloway

# CONTENTS

INTRODUCTION ..................................................................7

WHAT DO YOU NEED TO KNOW? ...............................9

CHOOSING A PEDIATRICIAN....................................... 11

*Does the pediatrician have a friendly personality and good communication skills?* .................................................................................... 11

*Are the staff good?*............................................................. 12

*Is the pediatrician well recommended?*........................... 12

*How is the location?* .......................................................... 12

WHAT TO EXPECT THE FIRST DAYS HOME .......... 13

*The Time Factor*................................................................. 13

*Relationship Strain* ........................................................... 14

*Postpartum Depression*..................................................... 16

*Symptoms of postpartum depression include*..................... 17

*If you suffer from postpartum depression, try to beat it with the following:* ...... 17

*Postpartum Depression for Dad?*...................................... 18

*Siblings* ............................................................................... 19

*Conditions that may appear at birth – Don't be alarmed*............ 19

WHAT TO CONSIDER: ....................................................23

*Home healthcare*................................................................. 23

*Establish a support system* ............................................... 24

BREASTFEEDING.............................................................27

*Breastfeeding tips:*.............................................................. 28

*Reading the signs* .............................................................. 30

*Your milk flow too slow*..................................................... 31

*Your milk flow is too fast*.................................................. 31

*Burping*................................................................................ 32

*A successful feeding*.................................................................*32*

*What you should eat while breastfeeding*.........................*33*

*Timesaving Nutritious Meals:*.............................................*35*

*Foods to avoid when breastfeeding*......................................*36*

## BATH TIME! ........................................................................... **39**

*What you will need:*..............................................................*40*

*How to bathe a Baby* ............................................................*41*

*Tips for a successful baby bath*............................................*41*

*Sponge baths* ..........................................................................*42*

*Bath safety* .............................................................................*42*

## DIAPERING ........................................................................... **45**

*What you need* ........................................................................*46*

*Here's how it's done: How to change a diaper* .................*47*

*How often should you change your baby?*............................*48*

*Diaper rash*............................................................................*49*

*Helpful Hints:*.......................................................................*49*

*Cloth Diapers* ........................................................................*50*

## WHY IS MY BABY CRYING? ......................................... **51**

*Hunger*......................................................................................*53*

*Need for sleep*..........................................................................*53*

*A dirty diaper*.........................................................................*53*

*Colic* ..........................................................................................*53*

*Wants to be held/rocked*.......................................................*54*

*Too cold /Too hot*...................................................................*54*

*Needs to burp*..........................................................................*54*

*Teething* .....................................................................................*55*

*Sudden change in temperature*.............................................*55*

*Tight clothing* ........................................................................*55*

*No reason at all*......................................................................*56*

**YOUR BABY'S SLEEP**.................................................................**57**

    *Baby's sleeping area*................................................*58*

    *The right environment*.............................................*59*

    *Sleep Associations*...................................................*59*

    *What the experts say*................................................*59*

    *Parent-soothing method*...........................................*59*

    *Self-soothing method*...............................................*60*

    *Sleep tips*................................................................*61*

    *Which sleeping position is best?*................................*65*

    *Music for your baby's mood*.....................................*65*

**BABY'S DIET IN THE FIRST YEAR** ...............................**67**

    *What's on the Menu?*...............................................*69*

    *Ready-made baby food*.............................................*69*

    *Yummy fruits*..........................................................*69*

    *Cereal* ....................................................................*69*

    *Vegetables*..............................................................*70*

    *When can your baby eat yogurt?*...............................*70*

    *Mealtime Tips:*........................................................*72*

**YOUR BABY'S HEIGHT AND WEIGHT:**.........................**75**

    *What are growth charts?*..........................................*75*

**BABY TALK - LANGUAGE DEVELOPMENT IN YOUR CHILD**
.............................................................................................**77**

    *First Three Months*.................................................*78*

    *Months three through six*.........................................*80*

    *Six through nine months*..........................................*80*

    *Nine to twelve months* ............................................*82*

    *How to encourage language development*......................*82*

    *Language Delay*......................................................*83*

**TEETHING** .......................................................................... **85**

*Teething symptoms*.............................................................. *86*

*The Teething stages*.............................................................. *87*

*Caring for your baby's teeth* ................................................ *88*

**UNDERSTANDING YOUR BABY'S MOTOR SKILLS** ............... **89**

*What to expect?* ................................................................ *90*

*How to monitor and support motor skill development*........................ *91*

*How to monitor your baby's motor skills*...................................... *92*

**IMMUNIZATIONS** ................................................................. **95**

*Why are babies immunized?*.................................................. *96*

**Which vaccines do what?**................................................... *97*

*DTaP/IPV/Hib*............................................................... *97*

*Tetanus*......................................................................... *97*

*Polio* ............................................................................ *97*

*(Hib) Influenza type B*....................................................... *98*

*Whooping Cough*.............................................................. *98*

*Rotavirus vaccine Rotarix*.................................................... *98*

*Flu vaccine* ..................................................................... *98*

*MMR*........................................................................... *99*

*Overall*.......................................................................... *99*

**YOUR BABY'S FIRST COLD** ................................................. **101**

*How to treat a cold*............................................................ *102*

**CONCLUSION** .................................................................... **103**

# Introduction

Becoming a new parent is one of the most thrilling and life-changing experiences you'll ever have. If you are a first time mom or dad you're probably still experiences you're probably still trying to take it all in – the miracle of pregnancy, birth, and

Caring for a newborn is also one of the most daunting and challenging jobs you will ever take on. It's also one of the most exhausting. The seemingly endless cycle of feeding, diaper changes, trips to the pediatrician and sleepless nights you may mat leave feeling completely worn out and even wondering if it was all worth it. But seeing your baby smile at you for the first time, reaching out your hands to him as he takes his first steps, hearing him speak his first "mama" or "dada" will fill your heart with such indescribable joy and love, and you will feel that yes, it's all worth it, and more.

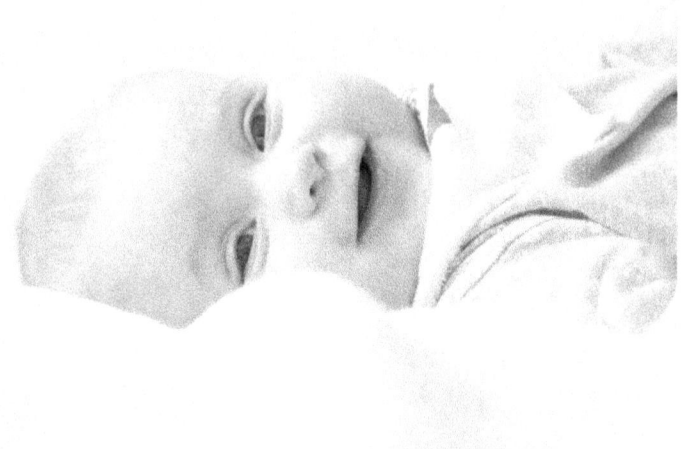

Caring for your baby during his first year is a lot of time and effort but that should not deprive you of enjoying being a new parent and spending many happy hours with your baby during this first wonderful year.

This book was designed to walk you through your new parenting responsibilities during your baby's first year. I hope the many tips and guidelines included here will show you that the task is not so daunting after all, and equip you with the skills and confidence to expertly care for your baby.

# What do you need to know?

Just a few decades ago, new mothers would spend from four days to a week in hospital. Today, many spend very little time in the hospital or birth center, usually going home the very next day. The hospital or birth center can't be relied on to give you the time or adequate information to care for your baby.

Newborn education classes can provide useful guidelines not all parents may have the time to attend them. Parents who do attend classes are still left worrying about whether they are doing everything right

Having this book on hand will hopefully help you fill in the gaps and deal with your bewilderment as a new parent. Most new parents generally have the same concerns regarding baby care. Most of these concerns have to do with everyday matters, such as childproofing a home, bathing the baby, monitoring development and so on.

To provide the best care for you baby and ensure his health and well-being, you also need to be well-informed on topics such as breastfeeding, sleep issues, introducing solid foods, buying baby clothes and gear, vaccinations and basically adapting your schedule to the new family member.

There can also be more serious concerns such as when to know your if baby is sick and needs to see the pediatrician, finding reliable and trustworthy daycare and nutritional issues.

The advice in this book has been drawn from current medical and expert recommendations from pediatricians to provide you with answers to essential questions and issues.

To sum up: Caring for a new baby is a true rest of resolve but also one of the most rewarding and joyful experiences life has to offer. This first year of your baby's like is indeed a year of many "firsts" – the first smile, the first tooth, the first step, and perhaps even the first panic rush to the doctor when there's nothing wrong!

# Choosing a Pediatrician

The health of your new baby will naturally be one of your biggest concerns and the first year will most likely have you making quite a few trips to the pediatrician. Having pediatrician who skilled accommodating and understanding is crucial, as you may have to contact him frequently over what will turn out to be false alarms – this is very normal with new babies especially. Ideally, you should search for and choose your pediatrician before your baby is born to avoid last-minute scrambles.

Here is what to look out for when choosing your pediatrician:

*Does the pediatrician have a friendly personality and good communication skills?*

Some pediatricians may be extremely good medically but not too good at personal skills. Their formal, their tight-lipped style tend to put of parents immediately A patient doctor who takes the time to listen to your concerns and explain exactly what the case is with your child is crucial for you at this stage.

## Are the staff good?

You can actually get a fair idea of what a doctor is like just from his office and staff. A comfortable, baby-friendly office and engaging staff are often signs that the doctor himself will be very accommodating to your needs.

I remember a certain pediatrician's office where the doctor was above and beyond great, however his staff were impossible. I once called the office because my child was sick and needed medication right away and the receptionist told me they could see my baby in three weeks. Shortly after, I found a new doctor.

Remember that you and your baby will be spending time baby will spend time with nurses, assistants and others, not just the doctor himself. They should be neatly-dressed, well-trained and supportive.

## Is the pediatrician well recommended?

The most common way people find good pediatricians is by word of mouth. Talk to friends and family members who have had first-hand experience ask them why they would recommend their pediatrician. Even so, you may have to go through a few hits and misses before you settle on the doctor that you feel is tight for you.

## How is the location?

You may want to consider this as factor, especially if you are a busy working mom, and also for unexpected emergencies. This should not be a top priority; don't settle for someone mediocre just because his office is in 5 minutes away, but again, don't choose a doctor in the next town.

# What to expect the First Days Home

## The Time Factor

From the minute you return home with your new baby, there's one thing you need to know: getting the hang of caring for your baby will be a 24/7 job in the first few weeks.

Becoming a parent a parent means your time is no longer your own. Deciding to go out to dinner or a move on the spur of the minute is no longer an option, especially more so with a newborn baby.

Any outings or travel plans will require a lot of planning, whether it's finding a baby sitter or even taking your baby along when you travel. The faster you adapt yourself to this reality, the easier it will be in the long run.

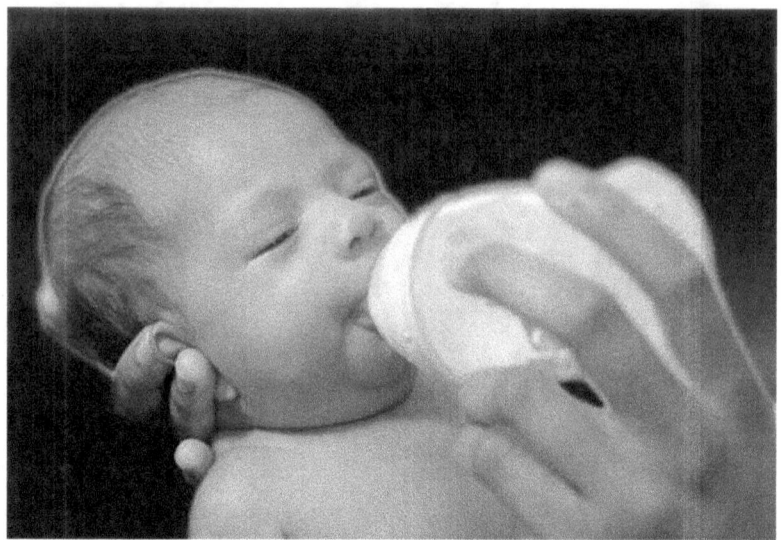

If you're a working mother you also need to arrange for appropriate childcare and if possible adapt your working hours around your baby. Many mothers will even trade fulltime jobs for part-tome ones or even give up working completely as they just can't bear to be away from their little ones for too long.

As long as you bear in mind that your baby comes first, you should be able to arrange your schedule according to your personal circumstances,

## Relationship Strain

A newborn baby can really test a couple's relationship and put immense pressure on it, more so if it's your first child. You'll feel that your whole day is spent on diapering, feeding, burping and rocking your baby to sleep. Even then, you may have to get up several a times during the night when your baby cries. The result: no time to spend with your partner.

It's a well-known fact that most men, being big babies themselves will often feel jealous of all the attention you're giving to the baby, as much as he is thrilled at being a dad.

It takes time to adjust to parenthood, and the best way to weather out this rather stressful time is to make dad an active participant in caring for the baby.

Some men are very hand-off when it comes to caring for babies – they just like to play with them! Talk your partner and tell him that you need and expect his help as it will be hard for you to do it alone. Many parents take turns changing diapers and getting up at night for the baby.

One couple I know actually alternated days when one spouse would sleep in the baby's room, quickly getting up to soothe or feed him when he cried, ensuring that the other partner got a full night's sleep.

It's quite natural that the hectic pace of day-to-day baby care will put a strain on any couple's relationship but this phase will quickly be over. Once adapt to your new roles as parents, you will have more time to spend together and nurture your relationship. Remember- you're in this together!

If you're parenting without a partner, you may feel pretty overwhelmed at first. Not having a partner to share in the work may leave you feeling exhausted and frustrated.

Establish a support system; having a supportive network of family and friends who can drop by to help you out, look after your baby or just listen, will help you immeasurably. For example, If your mother lives nearby, you can be sure she would love to drop in and look after her precious grandson/granddaughter while you enjoy a nap. or just listen to you will help greatly.

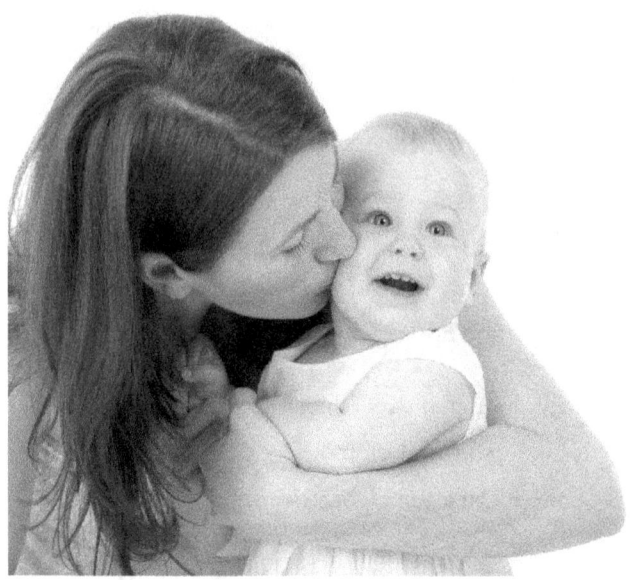

You might also consider joining a single mothers group. Not only are you sure to get a lot of emotional support, but swapping baby stories is always so much fun!

## Postpartum Depression

Emotional ups and downs are commonly experienced by both parents during the first weeks of their baby's life, but moms are especially vulnerable.

During this time which is called the postpartum phase, several factors come into play that make a woman more vulnerable to mood swings such lack of sleep, massive hormonal changes, and feeling overwhelmed can cause postpartum depression – or "baby blues"

Health experts say that almost all new mothers experience bots of postpartum depression in one form or another. For some, it can be in the form of very mild emotional fluctuations that usually subside in a week or two.

Eating healthy, exercising getting enough sleep are usually enough to rid you of baby blues. The help of supportive family and friends can also help get you over this phase quickly.

In some cases, however, the symptoms may be more serious and longer lasting, and may require treatment.

## Symptoms of postpartum depression include

- Feelings of overwhelming melancholy and sadness accompanied by crying fits.

- Constant exhaustion and listlessness, having little or no energy.

- Noticeable weight gain or weight loss.

- Feelings of guilt and worthlessness.

- Having no interest or concern for your baby.

*If you suffer from postpartum depression, try to beat it with the following:*

- Get as much sleep and rest relaxation as possible. Adapt your sleeping time to your baby's and sleep whenever he sleeps, or take advantage of this quite down to sit down and relax.

- Don't be too hard on yourself. Don't put yourself under pressure to "get back to normal" – relax, you will! Your body's been through a tough time and regaining your former figure and energy will not happen overnight.

- Enlist your family's help with housework and so on.

- Discuss your and compare your conditions with other mothers who experienced postpartum depression.

Try not to spend too much time alone when you're down – stay active in mind and body and don't surrender to gloomy thoughts - read an interesting book, call up a friend for a chat or go for a short, invigorating walk. Get professional help if your depression feels overwhelming or ongoing, or if those around you are concerned. Speak to your caregiver; he will advise you on what's best to do.

## Postpartum Depression for Dad?

A new dad does not experience the rollercoaster of hormonal and physical changes that a new mom does, yet he may also go through the male version of postpartum trauma. This is an assortment of emotions ranging from confusion, fear, and uncertainty to outright depression.

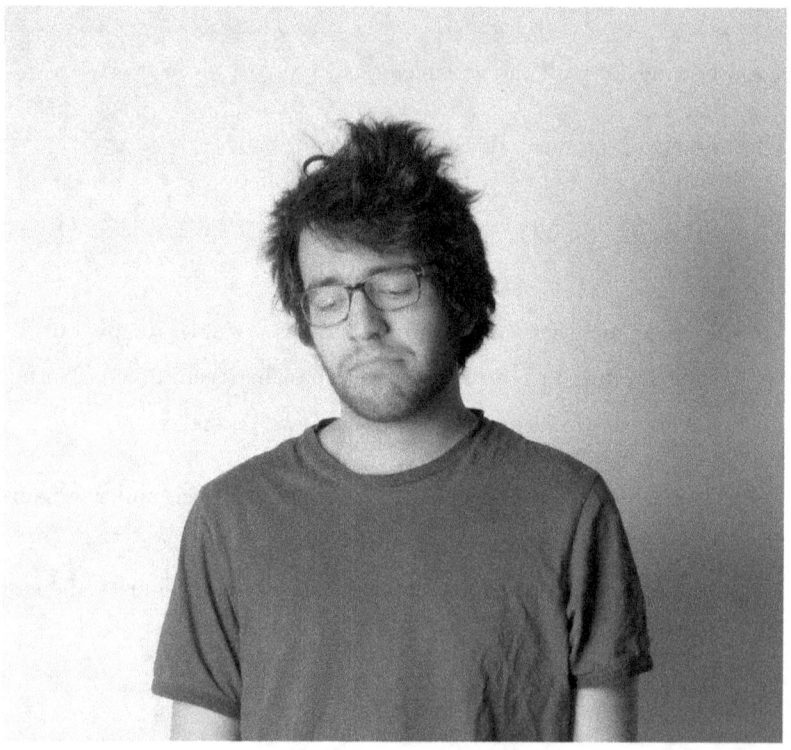

All of these emotions are a result of his new role as a dad, despite that fact that he is deliriously happy with the new baby and loves him intensely.

## Siblings

If you have an older child, you may have prepared him for the soon-to-arrive sister or brother. Even so, he may still have trouble accepting the fact that he is no longer the only child in the family.

The following symptoms are a clue that your child is suffering from sibling jealousy:

- Bedwetting

- Wanting to nurse from you

- Thumb-sucking

- Change in sleep patterns

There's no need worry at all. This regressive behavior is normal. Your child is afraid the new baby will take you from him and feels insecure.

Buy a gift your child will love and give it to him when he sees the new baby for the first time. Tell him his new baby brother/sister got it especially for him. If the child is young enough to not understand this little ploy, it'll work wonders.

Also, try to spend some one-on-one time with your child as much as you can. This will reassure him and make him feel that he is still very much loved. Listen to his feelings about his new sibling and discuss the pros of being an older child.

## Conditions that may appear at birth – Don't be alarmed

Even after a normal delivery without complications, a baby me be born with one or more of the conditions listed below. There is no cause for alarm as they will usually disappear over time.

**Birthmarks:** These are very common and can appear on various areas of the baby's body. They're completely harmless and will most likely fade or disappear completely by the time the child is five or six.

**Broken Collarbone:** This may occur as the baby is pushed out during a vaginal birth. This is not an uncommon condition and is not serious. You may see a little bump at the point of the break. In most cases no treatment is required the bone will heal very well on its own and the bump will disappear in a few weeks. All that's required is a little care when lifting the baby to spare him any discomfort.

**Dysplasia of the hips:** This basically means a displacement of the hip joint and is detected during the first days or weeks after the birth. Again, it will generally heal on it on without treatment. Your baby's caregiver will monitor the problem and advise if any treatment is necessary. The condition is more common in girls and babies who were in a breech position.

Bruised scalp or elongated head: Bruising is due to the baby's head pressing against the mother's pelvic bone during birth during birth, causing blood vessels in the head to swell. An elongated head or hard bumps on the scalp may occur when suction or forceps are used to deliver the baby. Remember, the bones in a newborn's head are still very soft. No need to panic – both these conditions disappear completely within the first one or two weeks.

**Heat Rash:** This is common in hot climates. The rash appears in the form of tiny red pimples in the folds of the skin and on the baby's face and neck. This is easily treated with cool sponge baths, baby powder and by keeping your baby dry and cool.

**Jaundice:** This condition is also quite common and is easily detected when your baby is examined after birth; it is commonly detected through a yellowish tinge to the baby's skin. Baby jaundice is easily treated and is rarely serious. It occurs because the baby's immature liver has not yet begin to function to full capacity.

**Sacral Dimple:** You may notice a large shallow dimple at the base of your baby's spine just at the top of the buttocks. Again this is no cause for concern and will fill our over time. In rare cases, it may be a cause for a more serious spinal condition. Your health practitioner will advise you if further evaluation is needed.

**Diaper rash:** This is by far the most common problem with newborns because their skin is so sensitive. Using organic wipes and diaper rash creams will help soothe the rash. If your baby baby's rash is excessive you should consider switching to cloth diapers. Diaper rash is nothing serious but does cause a lot of discomfort to a baby so be extra diligent in keeping him dry.

# What to consider:

## Home healthcare

Because the majority of mothers today go home very shortly after their delivery, some parents are now opting for home health care, where a healthcare professional will come in at arranged times to check on the baby's health

Postnatal issues such as jaundice, feeding, umbilical cord and skincare are reasons why some parents feel it would be more beneficial to have home healthcare during the first week or two.

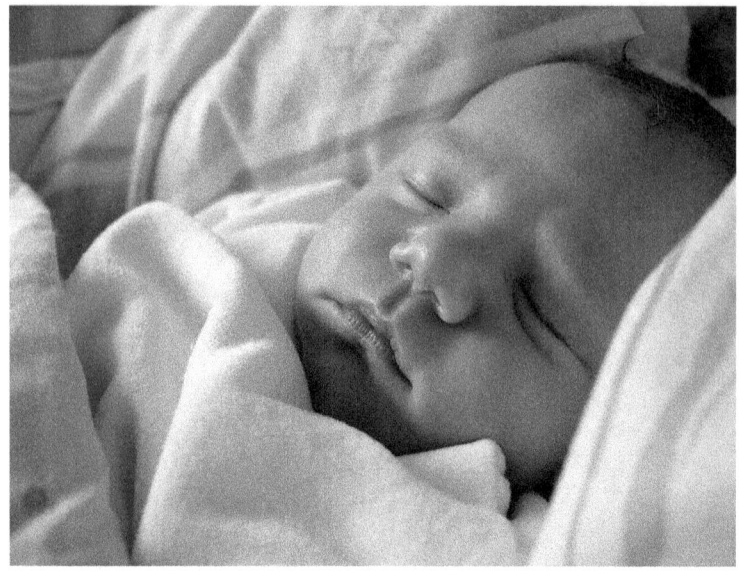

If you think you'll like some professional postpartum support, consider arranging a home healthcare visit shortly after you arrive home from the hospital or birth center. Usually, it is a nurse with newborn care training who will come to your home to examine and care for your baby and inform you if further medical care is required, First time mothers may also seek the help of a lactation consultants who can come to your home and advise you on breastfeeding.

If your baby is premature or has specific heath issues make sure your home care practitioner is informed about this beforehand as your baby will need extra monitoring.

Ask your doctor or hospital how this can be arranged and check if your health insurance plans covers he costs, as some plans do cover home care.

## Establish a support system

This is very important for new or single mothers. The physical and emotional changes that accompany childbirth and the huge responsibility of caring for a newborn may understandably leave you feeling overwhelmed.

The added responsibility of having to work, cook and keep the house cleaned plus make sure your baby is well cared for is an added pressure.

You DON"T have to do this alone! A good support system will not only ease the pressure immensely but will also give you time to enjoy these first wondrous weeks with your child.

Don't be afraid to ask. You'll find that friends, parents and even neighbors will generously and eagerly help out with a dozen chores like cooking a meal to cleaning the house, running errands and babysitting while you rest, nap or go for a walk they will also be generous with emotional support and encouragement, a great way to quickly get over those baby blues.

**Tip:** Make a mental list of the kinds of help you need and who can best provide it. For example, a neighbor who picks up her kids from school every day can stop at the grocery store and pick something up for you. Don't be hesitant to ask; you'll be pleasantly surprised at how eager people will be to help.

**Types of help you may want to consider:**

- Household chores such as cooking and laundry.

- Transportation to doctor's appointments.

- Baby care such as bathing or feeding.

- Babysitting while you take a quick nap, walk or shower.

- Errand to the grocery store and pharmacy

- Companionship.

- A sympathetic shoulder to cry on!

ELANE HOLLOWAY

# Breastfeeding

Science has proven that breast milk is by far the best nourishment for your baby during this crucial period of development and boosts natural immunity to many diseases. It also helps promote brain development. It has been found that babies who are bottle fed are more prone to childhood illnesses, and many more mothers today are opting to breastfeed their newborns because of the many proven benefits this entails.

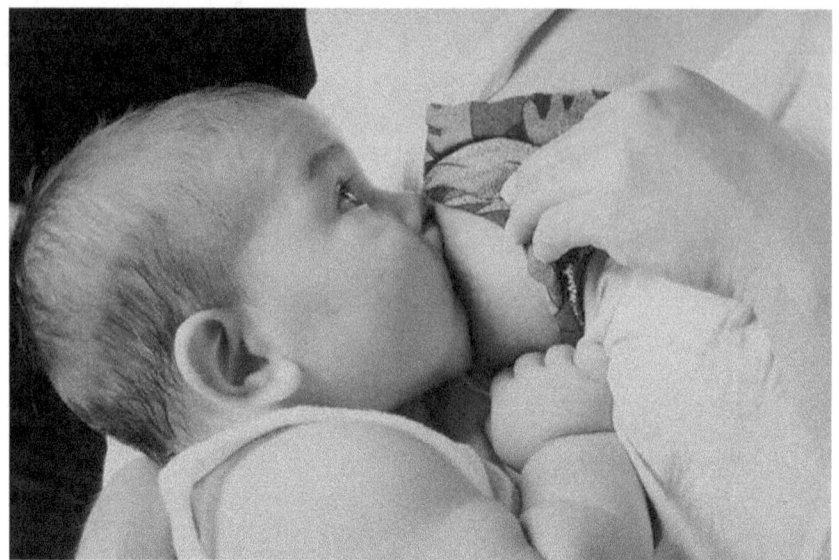

If you have chosen to breastfeed your baby, it is recommended that you nurse him as soon after birth as possible. The very first milk that flows from your breasts, called colostrum, is especially packed with natural antibodies that will immensely boost your baby's resistance to disease and give him the healthiest possible start. Don't worry if your breasts don't fill up with milk immediately. It usually takes 2 to 5 days for the colostrum to thicken, increase and turn into mature breast milk.

Some mothers worry that their baby may not be getting enough nutrition on breast milk alone - this is a fallacy. Breast milk is more than sufficient to sustain your child during the first months of his life. As long as the baby is gaining weight normally and does not seem fretful or hungry then your milk supply is sufficient. You can normally continue to breastfeed your baby for up to two months on breast milk alone as long as your milk supply is sufficient.

## Breastfeeding tips:

Nurse your baby frequently in the first few weeks to get your milk flowing and increase the supply.

Do not give your child water in a bottle or a pacifier as this will confuse him. Remember, your newborn is still learning to breastfeed and water does not flow as fast from a bottle, while nothing at all flows from a pacifier.

Your breast milk should be enough. A healthy newborn doesn't need water, juice or any other form of nutrition for least the first month

Vitamin D helps your baby absorb calcium and phosphorous which are important for strong, healthy bones. Your pediatrician may prescribe a supplement for your baby in case your breast milk does not contain enough.

Nurse your baby every two hours (including during the night) throughout the first month. Newborns tend to sleep a lot at first so it may be hard to stick to this schedule. If more than 2 hours have passed during the day and 4 during the night, wake your baby up to nurse.

Nurse your baby at the first sign of hunger such as fretting or sucking on his hands. You shouldn't wait for him to start crying.

Let you baby nurse for as long as he wants as long as he is actively sucking, taking time to alternate to the other breast. When the sucking subsides or your baby falls asleep then you know he is full.

Waiting too long between feedings will cause your breasts to engorge and feel uncomfortable, that's why you need to feed your newborn regularly, even at night.

Let your baby finish the first breast before moving him to the second.

To minimize the discomfort of full breasts between feedings, apply cold compresses.

If the baby has troubling latching on to you nipple because of engorgement, express some milk until the nipples is soft and try again.

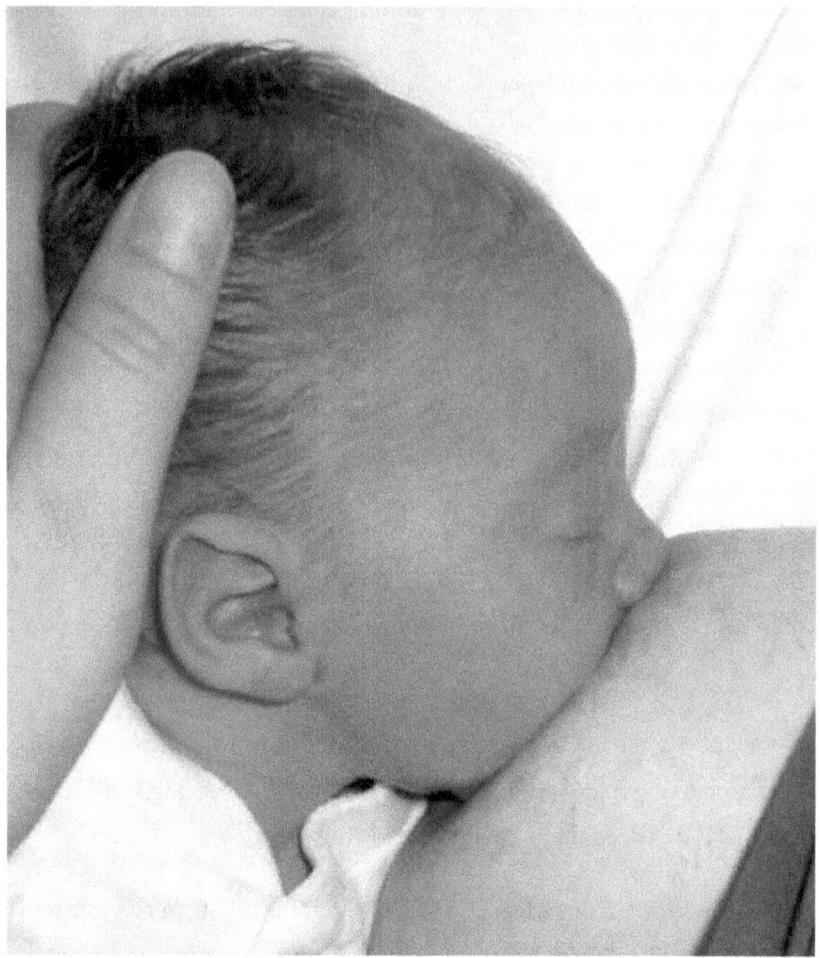

## Reading the signs

Breastfeeding seems like such a mystery. How can you tell if your baby is getting enough, too little or too much? Are you doing it right? Is your baby comfortable? Well… just ask your baby! Newborns have an astonishing ability to communicate if you just read the signs

A new born baby may seem such a mystery, but he or she does have a surprising ability to communicate and tell you exactly what is happening during breastfeeding.

**Look for the following signs:**

*Your milk flow too slow*

Your baby's eyes will be wide open, there will be long pauses between suckling or he may seem to be making little effort to suckle. He's telling you that your milk flow is too slow for him. Massaging the breast to increase the flow.

Another sign that your milk flow is too slow is that your baby falls asleep while nursing, with his mouth still firmly attached to the nipple. If you remove the baby, he will immediately start rooting and crying, trying to re-latch onto your breast. This is a sign that milk flow was so slow that your baby actually fell asleep while waiting for more.

If this becomes a problem ask your doctor's advice on how to improve your milk flow, as your frustrated baby may eventually reject the breast altogether.

Another sign that your milk flow is too slow is that your baby may suck and gulp eagerly for the first few minutes and then seems to slacken. If you have to keep stimulating your baby to suck, then your milk flow is probably too slow.

A baby who wants to suckle all the time, even right after feeding is telling you that he's still hungry.

*Your milk flow is too fast*

Your baby will nurse in quick noisy gulps and may even look a little bit startled! If this is the case then your flow is too fast and strong. Hold the baby as upright as possible (like in the above picture) so that the baby's throat is elevated above the nipple.

Also, is the baby still seems hungry after the first breast but cries when offered the second, again the milk flow from the second is too fast while the baby is still hungry.

The baby me appear to be swallowing well but his upper body is wriggling or he burps while nursing. This can also be a sign that the milk flow is too fast.

## Burping

Some babies just naturally burp in between sucking and continue nursing. This is normal and no cause for alarm.  Bur you should not interrupt a feeding to burp the baby unless he seems to be uncomfortable.

Always burp a baby after feeding to get rid of air that the baby has sucked in while nursing.

## A successful feeding

The breastfeeding experience is different for every nursing mother and child and there are really no fixed rules. However, it's important to establish a regular pattern once mature breast milk starts flowing around day 4 or 5. Don't wait for your baby to get too hungry and start to cry as it will be more difficult for him to calm down and latch on to the breast. You may delay a diaper change and feed the baby first if this is the case.

The baby may look a little frustrated for a few seconds, sucking eagerly, until the milk starts to flow, and then he will start swallowing steadily. He may pause briefly between sucking several times.

If your baby is nursing successfully, his body will be completely relaxed and his eyes may close – but he continues to suck and swallow steadily. Near the end, there will be longer pauses and shorter bursts of sucking.

When your baby is full he will abruptly pull away from the nipple and lie in your arms quietly, satisfied and content, or his mouth ay go slack and let go of the nipple or he may fall asleep. Some babies fall asleep with their mouth still fastened to your nipple. Gently disengage your baby as this is not a good habit for him to get into. If the baby screams when you disengage him from your breast then he is still hungry. Congratulations! You have completed a successful feeding! You can now burp your baby, change his diaper and put him down for a nap.

## What you should eat while breastfeeding

The saying "eating for two" during pregnancy is an old wives' tale but with regards to breastfeeding it's a fact. What you eat directly affects your breast milk, and a proper diet is

A proper breastfeeding diet is essential for producing rich, nutritious milk for your newborn.

One of the wonders of breast milk is that it can meet your baby's nutritional needs even when you're not eating perfectly.

You are also eating for two because your body as well needs a healthy diet during this very hectic time. Actually, your baby won't really be harmed if you have a poor diet because mother's milk already contains all the nutrients he needs – it's you who will suffer more. Poor diet will force your body to draw on its reserves which will affect your energy and stamina – and you need every bit and more to care for your new child!

A healthy, balanced diet is essential for a breastfeeding mom, give or take the occasional lapse. Here are some guidelines to follow:

Drink lots of liquids, especially fruit juices to keep your milk replenished

Many moms feel extra hungry while breastfeeding which is logical, as your body is working non-stop to produce milk for the baby. The trick is to eat small main meals with healthy snacks in between to satisfy your hunger and keep your energy levels up. Keep your hunger in check and your energy level high.

If you were taking prenatal vitamins, you can continue to take them for extra energy, but they are not a replacement for nutritious food.

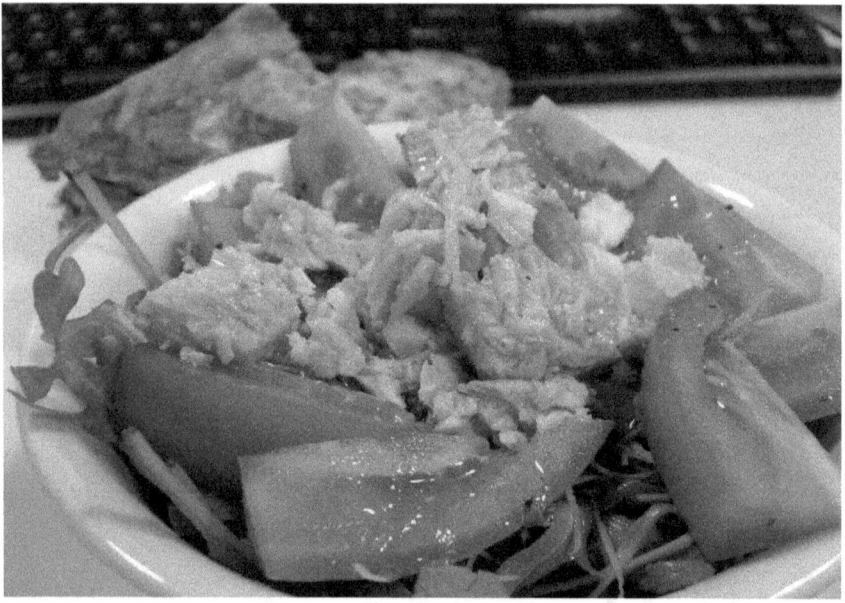

Foods to focus on are iron-rich foods and foods high in fiber. These foods will help keep up your strength while you're breastfeeding. To follow are the top 5 best foods for breastfeeding moms:

| FISH | A great source of high quality protein, and calcium, especially sardines and salmon |
| --- | --- |
| AVOCADO | Avocadoes are rich in folic acid, which your newborn needs for proper growth, and also a great source of vitamins C and E. |
| RED MEAT | Lean beef and lamb are one of the best foods for nursing mothers. Meat is high in protein, iron and B12, an important vitamin for your baby's neurological development. |
| LEGUMES | All types of beans, lentils and black eyes peas are very high in fiber and also contain iron and zinc |
| NUTS | Very high in nutrition and packed with Omega-3 fatty acids, protein and iron and are great energy boosters. |

## Timesaving Nutritious Meals:

I know, caring for a new baby is total time and energy-consuming and unless you're lucky enough to have a personal chef, meal preparation is just not a priority for you at this time. But making healthy eating a part of your lifestyle is no harder than popping a frozen meal into the microwave.

**Check out these tips:**

- Add a handful of fresh berries and nuts to your breakfast cereal or toss some dried fruit and granola into low-fat yogurt – instant energy!

- Add beans, peas and tuna to a lunch or dinner salad.

- Always have cut-up and prepared vegetables in zip-lock ready in the fridge. These can be steamed, eaten raw as a snack or added to salads.

- Add a spoonful of honey to yoghurt for an instant pick-me-up, and use honey instead of sugar in herbal teas.

- Add diced fresh fruit to yogurt for a healthy dessert or snack

- For a healthy protein-punch, keep some hard-boil eggs in the fridge. Slice them on top of a salad or simply grab one for a quick and filling snack.

- The trusty peanut butter sandwich is always a classic. Have a peanut butter sandwich on whole-grain bread topped with a spoonful of honey – it's fast, filling and will keep you going for hours. -

- Keep an assortment of fresh fruits on hand for quick snacks between meals. Bananas especially are extremely nutritious and filling. Apples are also great standby as they're available year-round.

Remember to drink lots of water to keep your energy levels high. Don't wait until you're thirsty. Regular water intake is important otherwise you may feel tired and nauseated. A glass of milk or juice is also fine but should not completely replace your water intake.

*Foods to avoid when breastfeeding*

Some foods can have a negative effect on breast milk or induce an adverse reaction of your newborn, therefore, you should stay away from the following:

- Strong herbs or spices, especially chili.

- Fish that may have high mercury levels, such as mackerel, shark and swordfish.

- Chocolate

- Citrus fruit

- Alcohol should be avoided altogether.

- Garlic

- Supplements unless with the permission from your doctor and cigarettes should be avoided by nursing mothers. Cigarettes especially reduce breast milk production and can cause vomiting, diarrhea and nervous tension in newborns.

# Bath Time!

Bathing your baby for the first time may be a frightening experience newborn, you may find it a little scary at first. Handling a tiny, slippery, wet newborn who will probably scream at the top of his lungs is a pretty intimidating task for any new parent. Stay calm; all it takes is a firm grip and a little practice.

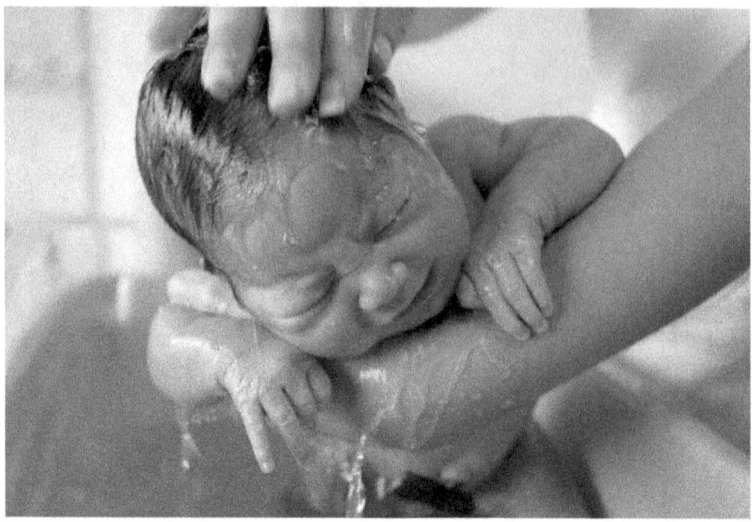

## What you will need:

Make sure all your supplies are at your fingertips. You do not want to run across the house with a wet naked baby in your arms to fetch something you've forgotten.

- Two cotton washcloths. One for the face, another for the scalp.

- Two soft towels. One can be hooded.

- Special baby soap or mild unscented soap.

- Baby shampoo – if your little one has hair!

- Cotton balls

- Baby lotion or diaper cream if needed.

- Fresh diaper and clothes

- A blanket to swaddle the baby if you are going to dress him in another room

# How to bathe a Baby

1.  The bath area should be a flat surface like a kitchen counter, table or even the floor, but the kitchen sink is fine, too. A small baby tub should be used. Do not bathe your baby in a regular tub as he is still too tiny and fragile.

2.  Fill the tub with about 3 inches of warm water. Test the water with your wrist and not your hand to make sure it's not too hot.

3.  Gently place the baby in the bath feet first while supporting his head and neck with one hand.

4.  Lay the baby in the water, keeping his head supported.

5.  Begin by washing that baby's face with a warm washcloth, gently cleaning the eyes and around the nose.

6.  Spa the washcloth and gently clean the baby's scalp.

7.  Scoop water over the child's body and lather him gently with baby soap from top to bottom, scooping water over him regularly to keep him warm.

8.  Rinse your baby thoroughly with clean warm water you have prepared in a bowl nearby.

9.  Wrap the baby snugly in a soft towel and pat him dry.

## Tips for a successful baby bath

Make sure you have everything you need within reach: towel, soap, change of clothes, baby lotion, etc.

Over-bathing may dry out a baby's sensitive skin. Bating a baby 3 times a week during the first year is sufficient.

Some babies love baths and find the warm water soothing. Other's scream incessantly – grin and bear it.

A bath should not take longer than 5 minutes as the water will start to cool.

Make sure there are no drafts as you move your baby from the bathing area to another room.

Don't bather your baby right after a feeding or when he's hungry.

## Sponge baths

It's best to stick to sponge baths for the first week or two until the baby's umbilical cord falls off and the area heals completely. Wash your bay with a washcloth sipped in warm water. In addition, remember to was his face and hands thoroughly frequently in between sponge baths.

## Bath safety

Never leave your baby unattended even for a second. If you absolutely must answer the doorbell or phone, wrap him in a blanket and take him with you.

Always fill the tub before placing your baby in it. Running water may get too hot.

Always test the water with your wrist. It should be just warm to the touch. A baby's skin is very fragile and can actually scald if the water is too hot.

This one is so important I'm going to repeat it: NEVER leave your baby unsupervised! A newborn can very quickly (within 60 seconds) drown in just one inch of water.

Keep your baby's head well supported and his upper boy well above the water.

Babies are slippery when wet! Be very careful when taking him out of the bath. If possible, have another adult standing by with the towel to take the baby from you.

Avoid using soap on the baby's face. If soap gets into your baby's eyes while you're washing his hair, just clean them with a damp washcloth.

ELANE HOLLOWAY

# Diapering

Changing diapers is not the most enjoyable part of baby care but sadly, you will spend quite a lot of your time doing this so you might as well learn how to do it efficiently - Especially as your baby may require as much as 10 or more changes a day!

Becoming an expert diaper changer probably wasn't on your list of future achievements but really, it does require quite a bit of skill.

Keeping your baby dry and comfy until he becomes potty trained is very important to prevent the dreaded diaper rash, which can cause him a lot of discomfort. With a little practice you will soon earn how to deftly and efficiently get through diaper changes and ensure that your little one is always dry and clean

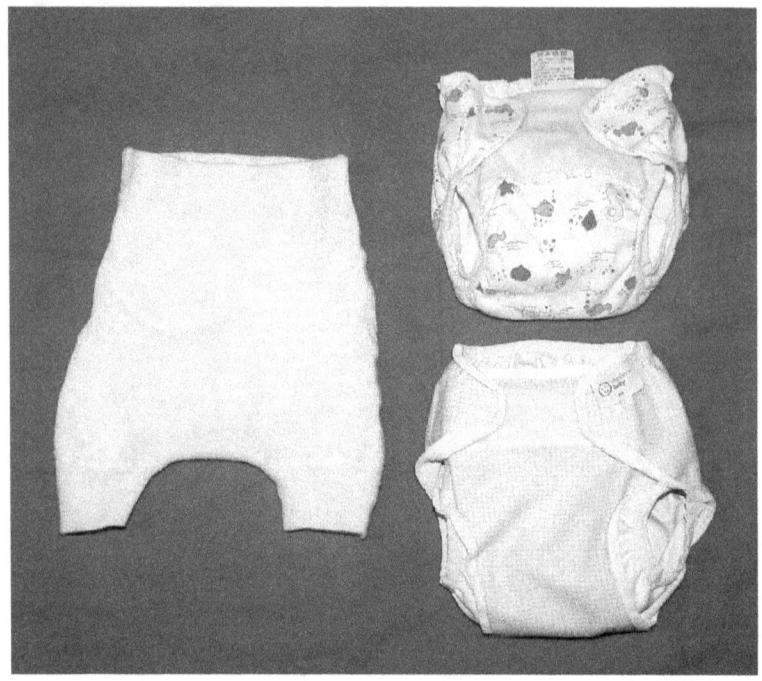

For some reason, dads especially see diaper changing as a mysterious, frightening and "icky" so if you're planning to enlist his help in this task, get him to practice with you and in a matter of weeks he too will become an expert!

## What you need

Make sure the following supplies are always on hand and remember to stock up regularly before the run out. There's nothing worse than having to run out for diapers at one in the morning!

- A clean diaper

- Wet wipes or a wet warm wash cloth. It's always recommended to use organic baby wipes or mild wipes for newborns.

- Rash cream (for use only when your baby gets diaper rash – they all do at some point)

- A suitable place for changing (changing table or bed)

- Changing pad to place under the baby if you are not using a changing table.

- Baby powder This is optional and can be used instead of rash cream or during every change just to keep your baby fresher.

- Baby lotion – this is also optional.

Before you begin, always make sure all your supplies are within easy reach. NEVER leave your baby unattended even for a second. be left unattended, even for a second. Newborns are surprisingly agile when it comes to rolling over, especially as the progress into the first few months.

## Here's how it's done: How to change a diaper

1. Spread out the fresh diaper, ready to use on the changing area.

2. Lay your baby down face-up.

3. Then unfasten the soiled diaper, gently lift the baby's legs up the ankles with one hand and with the other hand pull it out from beneath him.

4. Quickly fold the soled diaper over and lay it to the side or in a special bin you have near the changing table.

5. Thoroughly clean the baby's genitals and buttocks gently with baby wipes or a soft washcloth dipped in warm water.

6. Dry the area thoroughly with a burp cloth or soft, absorbent towel.

7. Apply baby lotion or sprinkle on baby powder cornstarch powder.

8. While lifting the baby's legs again with one hand, slip the clean diaper underneath him with the other fasten the tabs. The diaper should be snug but not too tight; you should be able to slip your fingers inside the diaper around the tummy.

## How often should you change your baby?

It's advisable in the first week or two to check your baby frequently and change him when necessary until you familiarize yourself with his needs or basic "schedule." Some babies require only a few diaper changes a day while others require much more doe a variety of reasons.

Generally, you will find that your baby needs changing at the following times:

- First thing in the morning: most babies will be quite wet in the morning unless you were able to change his diaper during the night . Even if the baby's hungry, change him first , even if you'll have to change him again after he eats to avoid diaper rash, which is more uncomfortable for your baby than a few hunger pangs

- Before bedtime. Never put your baby to bed with even a mildly wet diaper. A baby will fall asleep faster and sleep more confortable if he's clean and dry.

- During the night, probably once or twice especially during the first weeks when you have to get up for night feedings anyway.

- Always put on a fresh diaper after your baby's bath.

- After meals. Babies commonly have a bowel movement 20 – 45 minutes after a meal, and your newborn will let you know it in no uncertain terms – he will strain, his face will get red and in some cases you will even hear the movement being passed.

Remember that each baby is different, though, so learn to recognize your baby's signals and adapt your own pattern according to his needs. Just remember the golden rule: A clean bottom makes for a more cheerful baby!

## Diaper rash

As mentioned earlier, all babies do get diaper rash at some point and it's a very common – actually, it would be very uncommon id a baby did not get diaper rash during the first year.

Diaper rash appears on a baby's genitals, buttocks and thighs. It may appear as a slight redness or in the form of raised red areas around the thighs and genitals.

Change your baby more frequently than usual to keep the area as dry as possible. Cleanse well with baby wipes and use baby ointment or powder. If the rash is sever and keeps flaring up your pediatrician may advise you to switch to cloth diapers.

After changing and cleaning your baby, leave him without the diaper for a while as often as you can. This will deep him drier and help the rash heal faster – and your baby will absolutely love the feeling of not being confined in a diaper!

Diaper rash is not serious but it can make you baby very uncomfortable and irritable. It doesn't NOT mean that you are a negligent mother. As I said before it, would actually be very uncommon if babies did not get diaper rash at some point.

*Helpful Hints:*

Always wash your hands thoroughly after changing a diaper and use a hand sanitizer afterwards.

When changing a boy, wear some sort of shield such as plastic apron to protect you from unexpected "accidents." Keep your face well out of range as well!

As your baby gets older, he will tend to squirm and struggle more. Give him something to hold as a distraction to keep him lying still.

When cleaning your baby with wet wipes, always make sure to wipe gently from the front to the back to avoid spreading bacteria that can cause infection. This is especially important with baby girls. Make sure you also clean between the folds.

Never fasten the diaper too tightly. It should be snug but comfortable for your baby. You should be able to easily slide your fingers into the front of the diaper.

Never leave dirty diapers lying around. Dispose of them immediately in a covered bin and make sure the bin is emptied and sanitized regularly – this is especially important hen your baby begins to crawl.

*Cloth Diapers*

Some parents prefer to use cloth diapers as they are more environmentally friendly. Many parents also believe they are a healthier option for the baby.

Cloth diapers have certainly come a long way from the ones we once wore as babies; they are more absorbent, some come in two or three layers, some re pre-folded and some even com with Velcro strips so there's no need for safety pins. Cloth diapers may mean extra work though as you will have to wash them at home or sign up for a diaper service that will pick up the dirty diapers and deliver clean ones.

A cloth diaper is basically changed the same way as a disposable diaper. Pre-folded are the most commonly used and the most convenient

# Why is my baby crying?

New born babies cry a lot, sometimes for no apparent reason. A baby who cries frequently is one of the most common causes of worry and frustration for parents – what's my baby trying to tell me? Why does he cry so much? What could be bothering him?

When your baby is wailing, red-faced, kicking and pummeling his little fists in the air, chances are it's probably for one of the reasons below. Go down the list until you pinpoint the cause and are able to soothe your baby:

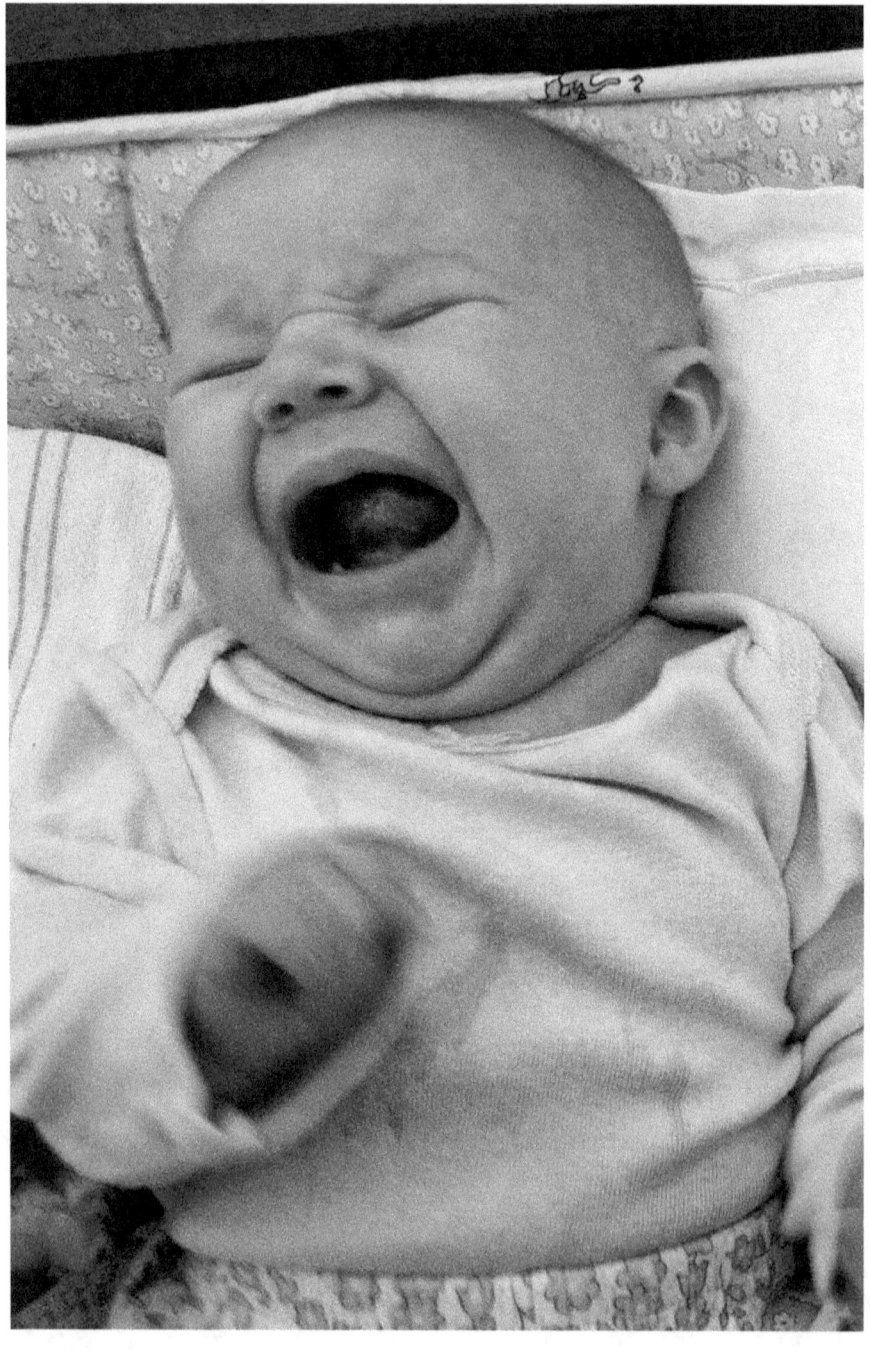

# Hunger

This is first thing you need to check when your baby won't stop crying. Some signs of hunger include putting has hands in his mouth and sucking the fingers, kicking and "rooting". Rooting is a reflex where the baby turns his head towards your hand if you stroke its face and makes suckling movements with the lips. A full belly quiet the crying and make you baby drowsy.

# Need for sleep

Babies can get very fussy and irritable when they need to go to sleep. You'd think that a baby can just fall asleep time but it's more common for them to fuss, cry and raise hell before finally settling down and nodding off. I call this the "sleep tantrum."

Babies tend to cry when they're overly tired as well so it's recommended that you stick to a naptime schedule and make sure your baby gets enough rest.

# A dirty diaper

Some babies are very finicky and will let you know immediately in no uncertain terms that their diaper needs changing. Others can tolerate a dirty diaper a bit longer. In either case, the baby will stop crying once he's clean and dry again.

# Colic

Colic is a mysterious condition associated with tummy troubles and gas and can lead to seemingly incessant crying during the first month or so. A baby with colic can cry nonstop for up to three hours a day for several days a week for up to 3 weeks.

If your baby is frequently fussy and cries right after being fed, it may be due to gas or stomach pain associated with colic. Many parents swear by the famous Gripe Water, a colic remedy that contains sodium bicarbonate and herbs. Get your doctor's okay before using this or any other over the counter baby gas remedy.

## Wants to be held/rocked

Crying can be your baby's way of telling you that he needs a cuddle. Babies love to be held close by their parents, to see their faces and hear their voices, and to even fell their heartbeats as they are being rocked.

You may wonder if too much holding or cuddling will spoil your baby – no. During the first few months it's actually advised to hold, rock, sing and talk to your baby as much as possible.

Naturally, you can expect our arms to ache a lot during this period, so you can alternate holding with carrying your baby around in a front carrier or sling. Your baby will still feel close and cuddled and your arms will get a much-needed respite!

## Too cold /Too hot

When your baby feels too hot or cold his natural response will be to quite vocal about it. If he cries when you remove his clothes to change a diaper, you can be sure it's because he feels chilly.

Newborns enjoy being bundled up and kept quite warm as a rule, but they will cry if they feel too warm. But babies are less likely to cry when the feel to warm that they are if the feel cold.

## Needs to burp

Babies feel a lot of discomfort when there is air in their stomachs. They are bound to swallow when he breastfeed or nurse from a bottle, and this air needs to be released by burping the baby. Hold the baby over your shoulder, taking care to support his back and gently massage or pat the middle of that back with the other hand.

Some babies are really uncomfortable when they have air in their tummy and need to be burped after every meal while others don't seem to require much burping.

## Teething

Your baby's first tooth will appear sometime between 4 and 7 months. The process of the tooth pushing out through your baby's tender gums can be painful, and he will cry and fuss a lot during this time and may run a low fever. Once the new tooth breaks out he excessive fussing and crying ill stop almost immediately after.

If your baby cries excessively and seems to be in pain, gently run your finger along his gums. If you feel the nub of a baby tooth under the surface, you'll have located the problem. Your baby's first tooth is about to appear!

Your pediatrician may prescribe a gum cream to numb the pain, or you may give your baby a teether to bite on – and no, it will not make your baby's teeth come out crooked. That's just an old wives' tale.

## Sudden change in temperature

Babies may cry when exposed to sudden hot or cold temperatures, such as when you're changing his diaper or bathing him. Some babies scream murder when they're being bathed the first few times but they soon grow to enjoy their bath-time

## Tight clothing

Make sure your baby's diaper is not too tight and that his clothing not too tight in certain areas such as around the neck, stomach or thighs.

# No reason at all

If you've checked off all the above possibilities and your baby is younger than 5 months old and still cries a lot, then he's simply doing it for no reason! A lot of babies seem to cry a lot in the late afternoon and early evening or no apparent reason and this is totally normal. Maybe they're bored, maybe they just like the sound of their own voice… who knows what goes on inside a baby's head at that age!

If your baby has a pattern of crying or no apparent reason, try the following:

- Hold your baby and pace around the room while rocking him.

- Sit with your baby in a rocking chair. Babies love the soothing rhythm of being rocked and will usually quiet down and fall asleep.

- Give him a warm bath.

- Gently rub his tummy or back.

- When your baby is old enough:

- Put him in a pushchair and take him for a walk

- Rock him gently in a baby swing.

- Give him something to suck on.

I won't mince words here. A baby's frequent or incessant crying can really drive parents up a wall. Frayed nerves may lead to loud arguments between spouses about whose turn it is to pick up the baby and rock him, and tempers can be very short indeed. It' a tough time but be sure that as the baby grows he will learn to communicate his needs to you in different ways and the crying will stop.

# Your baby's sleep

Newborns spend a lot of their time sleeping during the first few weeks. The problem is that they sleep in bursts of an hour or two and wake up crying – or need to be awakened to eat and be changed. A newborn's sleep pattern can really take its toll on parents but it it's not something you can enforce, so be prepared to be awakened at all hours of the night. The best you can do is provide a comfortable and quiet sleeping environment for your child where he can drift off to sleep without too much fuss.

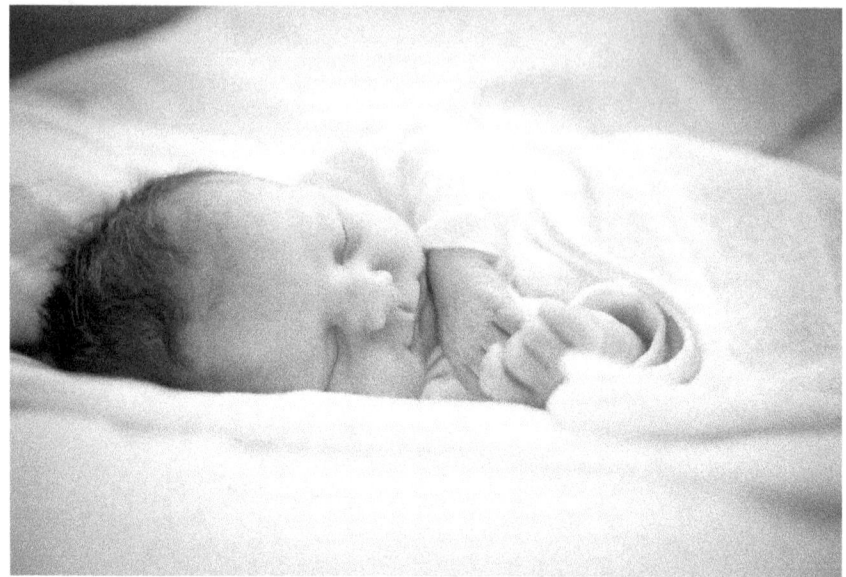

# Baby's sleeping area

There is no right or wrong place for a baby to sleep. Decide what works best for you in the first few months until your child settles into a regular sleeping pattern. Some parents keep the baby's crib in their own bedrooms for easier access when getting up throughout the night. Others prefer a separate nursery.

Sleeping arrangements depend a lot on your baby, too, and where you find he sleeps best. Some newborns sleep well in their own rooms, other sleep best in a crib or bassinet next to parents' bed, while others prefer to sleep right next to mommy in her bed.

Many parents arrange a "co-sleeper" arrangements where they take turns sleeping in the baby's room, allowing the other partner to get a good night's rest.

Sleeping arrangements will change as your child grows and may go from the child sleeping in your bed to sleeping in his crib, to finally sleeping through the night in his own room… yes, there is hope in sight!

*The right environment*

Your baby must drift off to sleep naturally and without too much fuss. It's your role to provide an environment conducive to sleep and teach your baby certain cues to let him know that he is expected to sleep.

*Sleep Associations*

Experiment with this method to find what works best, and alternate them throughout the first few months of your baby's development. You may find that what doesn't work best one week may work the next.

An infant will associate going to sleep with certain actions on your part such as rocking or singing and will quickly learn to fall asleep when these actions are performed. For example, if you nurse your baby to sleep, he will quickly associate nursing with sleeping.

Get your baby used to several sleep associations and alternate them, these can include, nursing, rocking, singing, even playing soft music or sitting with the child in a rocking chair.

## What the experts say

There are two schools of thought on the best way to put babies to sleep: the parent-soothing method and the self-soothing method. Both methods have their pros and cons.

*Parent-soothing method*

This is when the parent assists the baby to make a calm transition into sleep by nursing, rocking, singing, etc.

**Pros:**

- The baby learns a healthy sleep attitude by associating it with something that is calm and soothing, and a pleasant, safe state to be in.

- Builds fond memories of being lovingly parented and a stronger sense of security.

- Increases trust and bonding between parent and child.

**Possible cons:** The child may associate sleep with the presence of a parent and come to rely on this, putting an added burden on parents.

### Self-soothing method

This is where the baby is laid down and left to fall asleep on his own. Parents may offer some intermittent comfort but do not assist the child to drift off into sleep.

**Pros:** The baby learns to fall sleep by himself without reliance on the parent or associating parental comforting with sleep. Some may regard this method as somewhat tough on the baby but much less exhausting for parents.

**Possible cons:**

- Involves a few heart-wrenching nights of letting your baby "cry it out".

- Does not work for high-strung, high-need or with strong-willed babies – and babies are much more stubborn that you think. If your child is this type, he will wear you out with incessant screaming. It may be easier on your nerves to simply soothe him to sleep.

- In learning to ignore a baby's crying, parents my overlook underlying medical conditions.

- May desensitize parents to their child's cries create trust and security issues.

In the end, it's up to you to find the method that works best for you and your family. The ultimate goal is to create a healthy sleep attitude in your child while being sensitive to his needs.

## Sleep tips

Try to settle into a consistent nap routine. Choose the times of the day when you are most tired, say, 11:00 a.m. and 4:00 p.m. Lie down with your baby at these times every day for about a week and take a nap with him. This will get your baby settled into a daily nap routine and allow you to get some much-needed rest. Arrange your household routine around these nap times, make sure the house is quiet and do not be tempted to do chores or get something done during this quiet time when the baby's asleep.

Babies who have a regular day nap routine are more likely to sleep for longer stretches during the night.

A warm bath or gentle massage may relax your baby and help him drift off to sleep faster – but beware as this may actually stimulate some babies. See how it works for you.

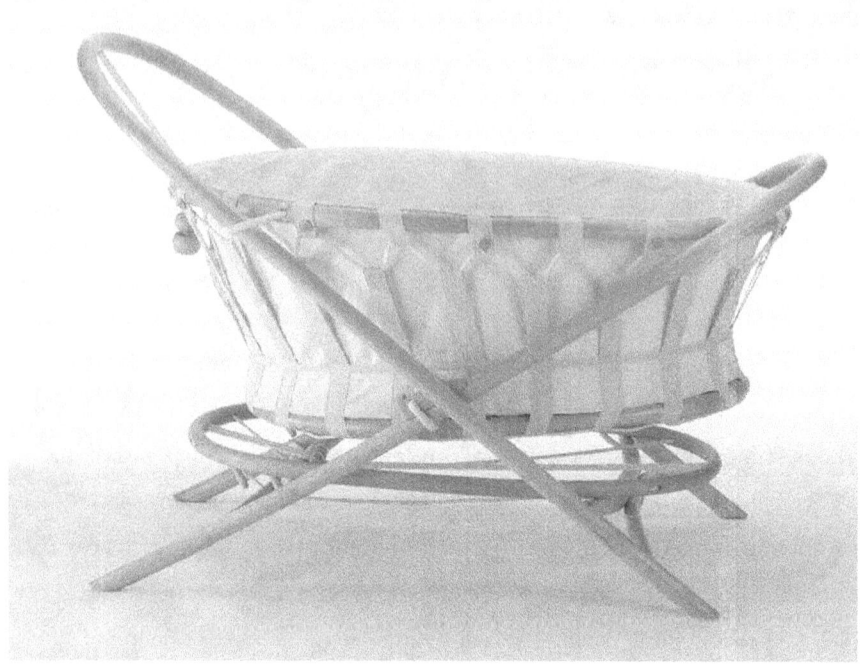

A tension-free, peaceful day will result in a restful night. The more you bond with your baby during the day, the more you hold and soothe and keep him calm, the more this peacefulness will carry through into the night.

Snuggling with your baby or nursing him before bedtime will create a feeling of warmth and security that is conducive to sleep.

A rocking chair may actually be a good investment at this time as it will relax your child before sleep while sparing you the effort of rocking in your arms or pacing. Cuddle your baby in your arms while rocking gently, singing or praying until he falls asleep.

If all else fails, a drive in the car may be the solution. Put the baby in a car seat and simply drive around until he falls asleep. HE will usually be in such a deep sleep when you return that you can carry the car seat with him in it to his room and leave him to finish his sleep.

Synthetic sleepwear may make some babies uncomfortable and restless. If you have gone through the whole repertoire of sleep inducing methods and still have trouble putting your baby to sleep, try cotton sleepwear.

For some babies, a wet diaper can be very uncomfortable and discourage sleep, while others may sleep through without any discomfort. If your baby can tolerate a wet diaper and is not suffering from diaper rash, it's better to let him sleep through rather than wake him up for a change.

A clear nose will help your baby sleep better, especially in the first month when babies breathe only through their nose. Bedroom inhalant allergies are a common cause of stuffy noses in newborns and can lead to frequent night waking. Keep your baby's room dust-free and remove any sources of lint such as fuzzy blankets and comforters, fuzzy toys, etc. If your baby is allergy prone, an air filter is a good investment – as well, the hum from the filter may even soothe your baby during sleep!

Teething pain is one of the main causes of sleep disturbance in newborns. Teething pain may start as early as three months and continue off and on all the way through two years, when the molars pus through. The signs that teething is the nighttime culprit are excessive drooling, tender gums, a slight fever and sometimes redness on the chin and cheeks. Get the okay from your doctor permission to give your child a dose of acetaminophen just before putting your baby to sleep.

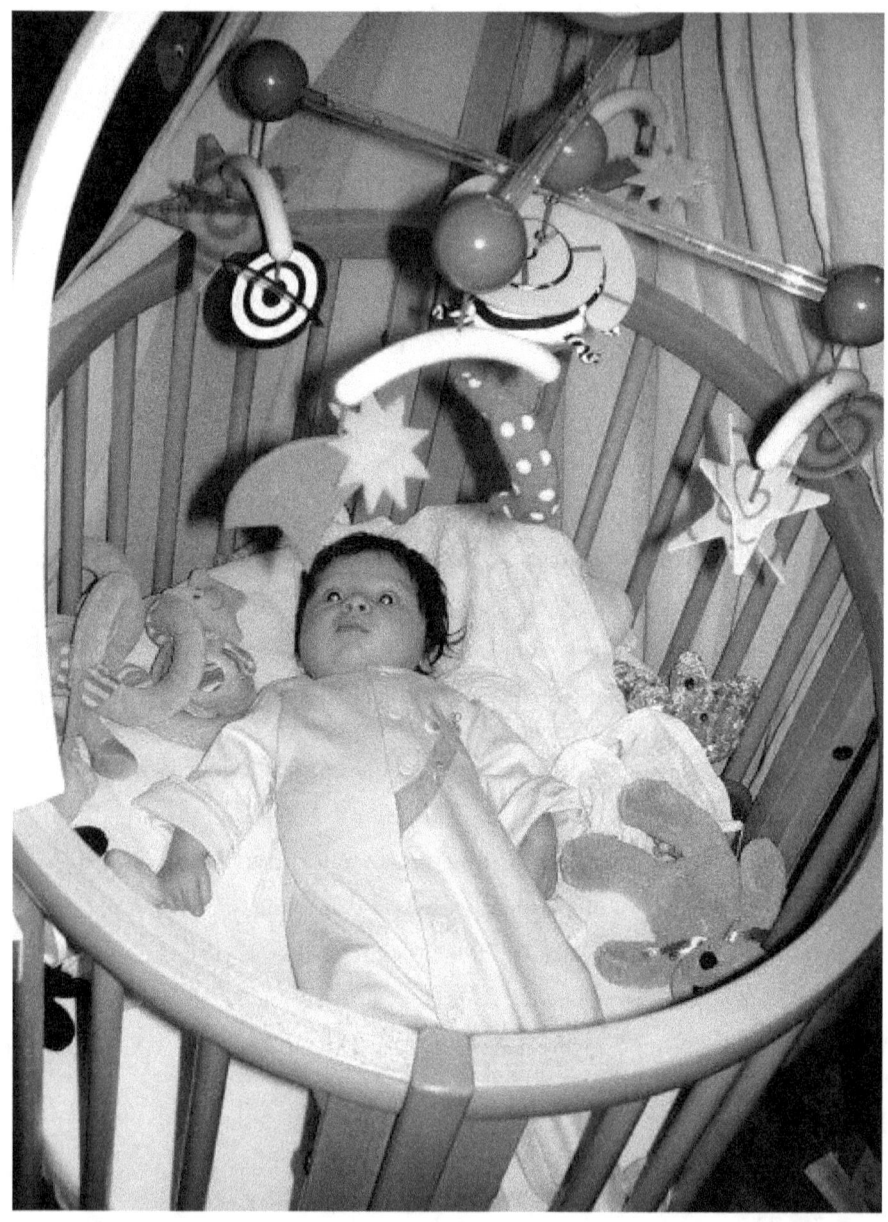

A warm bed is also conducive to restful sleep. Putting **a** warm, drowsy baby onto sold sheets can be trouble, especially when it's cold. Use flannel sheets or a warm towel for the baby's bed to make sure it's warm. The bedroom temperature should also be suitable, preferably kept at 70 degrees.

Playing recorded lullabies or nature sounds at bedtime and nap times is a great idea and very soothing for your baby.

When your baby wakes up during the night, do not move him to a brightly-lit room where there is noise or distraction such as a TV. change or feed him in his quiet room and soothe him back to sleep.

## Which sleeping position is best?

This is a hotly-debated topic on which there seems to be no agreement. Some experts say that placing the baby on his stomach is the ideal sleeping position as it prevent aspiration and helps him emit gas. On the other hand, recent studies seem to indicate that placing the baby on his back reduces the risk if SIDS (Sudden Infant Death Syndrome) but these findings are not conclusive. Proponents of the back position also say this helps the infant breathe better. The best advice I can give you here is to visit your pediatrician to discuss this matter.

## Music for your baby's mood

Do you sometimes listen to soft music when your stressed? Does listening to music make you feel good? Sure it does, and it will have the same effect on your baby. Music has a big effect on our moods, and some studies have shown that babies begin responding to music while still in the womb. We've all heard the theory that playing classical music for an unborn baby increases his chances of becoming a prodigy. In short, music can have a huge effect on your newborns mood and overall health.

Nature sounds, the hum of an air filter or vaporizer as well as music can calm even the fussiest babies. Playing music regularly for your baby even when he isn't crying will help associate the sounds with peace an calm.

Introduce your baby to music from day one – it's that simple and there's no right or wrong choice (except perhaps for heavy metal). There's no special song or ideal musical piece. Just play your favorite music whether it's classical music or pop and let baby enjoy with you.

In a few months, you will discover that your baby reacts to a certain song or piece, signaling that it's his favorite! Now you can play that song to him at bedtime or when he's irritable to soothe him – amazing!

# Baby's diet in the first year

From the time he's born until the age 4-6 months, your baby will get almost all of his nutrition from breast milk or baby formula. Liquids such as water and juice are gradually introduced and finally, solid foods.

The reason solid foods are not introduced earlier is to avoid your baby developing food allergies, and to ensure that he is old enough to "chew" and swallow well and will not choke.

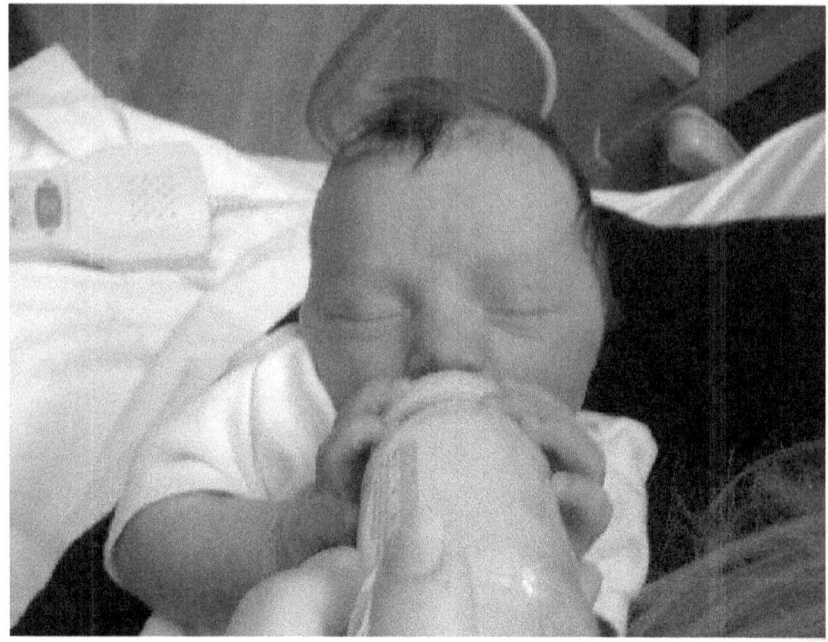

It's very important to note that not all babies are ready to start on solids at the same time and introducing ours to solids too early may makes him sick. What are the signs that your bay is ready?

**The following guidelines will give you that information:**

When your baby's birth weight had doubled. Liquids alone may not be sufficient at this stage to keep him satisfied and healthy.

The baby starts to show an interest in solids. If you put a dab of applesauce on his lips he will swallow it up eagerly and smack his lips, whereas before he may have puckered up his face.

When he can sit up with some support.

When he starts to frequently put things in his mouth.

When he is consuming 34 ounces of breast milk or formula daily.

This is the most important sing: Your baby always seems hungry!

Check with your doctor as well before you start your child on solids.

## What's on the Menu?

Regardless of what your child is going to eat, it needs to be super smooth and almost semi liquid.

### Ready-made baby food

It is nutritious and time-saving but if you are preparing your baby's food yourself, be sure to puree or mas and strain it so that it's almost falling off the spoon. You may add water as needed to reach this texture. As your baby becomes more experienced in eating solids, you may thicken the texture and refrain from adding liquids. This is usually at around 6 or 7 months.

**Note:** always introduce new foods one at a time and continue feeding them for 3-5 days to monitor if your baby has an allergic reaction.

Start with the three following foods:

### Yummy fruits

Fresh, mashed and strained bananas or baby food fruits such as apple sauce, peaches and pears. Your baby will love them and they are also highly digestible. I recommend you simply use jarred baby food as home preparation is just too much of a hassle.

### Cereal

Baby rice has always been recommend as the first food to introduce to a baby. It's nutritious, can be thinned or thickened as required and the bland taste will not put your baby off.

There are a variety of baby cereals on the market today and it's recommended you stick to one type (oat, barley or rice) at first. Avoid wheat cereals Avoid wheat cereals at the very start as it is an allergen.

Mix the cereal with breast milk, formula milk or boiled, clean water to create a smooth soup-like paste. Do not sweeten by adding applesauce, bananas or juice at this early stage.

*Vegetables*

Veggies are light, nutritious and not known to trigger allergies. Start with yellow or orange vegetables such carrots, sweet potatoes and potatoes. Save the green veggies for the next stage as your baby may find the taste too strong – Yes, from this age kids will start giving you a headache about eating their vegetables!

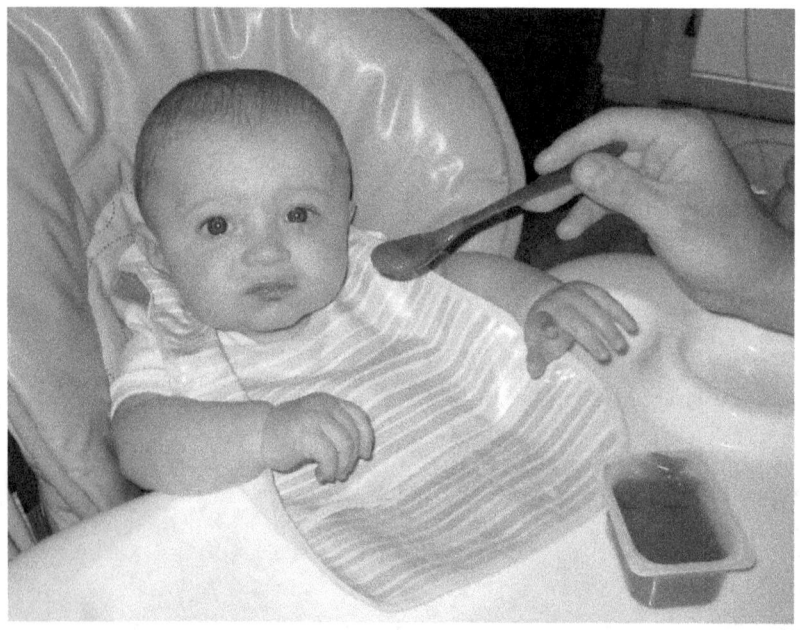

*When can your baby eat yogurt?*

You can give your baby plain, unsweetened yoghurt at around 6 months, after you have introduced him to other solids. Yoghurt is an excellent source of nutrition for your baby.

Why is it recommended to give your baby yoghurt but not cow's milk for the first 12 months? Cow's milk can make your baby iron deficient because a s a liquid, and easy for him to gulp down in quite a large amount. On the other hand, he's not likely to each a large enough quantity of yoghurt to make him iron deficient, while still getting enough milk protein.

**Note:** Cow's milk does not contain as much nutrition as breast milk or formula anyway so it's just naturally better to keep your baby off it for the first year.

Serve the yogurt plain or mixed with pureed fruit that you've prepared or baby food fruit that's sugar-free. This is one of the healthiest food combinations you can give your growing baby – but there are a few "buts":

Give your baby yoghurt once a day for three days straight so you can watch for an allergic reaction. If a red rash appears around your baby's mouth or he seems extra fussy or develops diarrhea, these are all signs of a food allergy. Check with his your pediatrician immediately.

Although very nutritious, yoghurt should not be a main diet feature in the first year, but a small part of a varied and healthy diet of other solid foods.

**NEVER** sweeten yoghurt with honey for the first year at least. Honey actually contains a bacteria that can cause botulism in babies.

**Don't** give your baby non-fat or reduced fat yoghurt before the age of two. He needs the fat and calories from whole-milk yoghurt.

**Don't** give your child flavored or fruit yoghurt as this almost always contains additives, artificial flavors and sweeteners. Adding fresh fruit to yoghurt is always the best option.

## Mealtime Tips:

Make mealtimes fun and enjoyable for your child so that he looks forward to eating his meals.

Always use a baby sip cup for juice and not a bottle. Juice in a baby bottle can cause dental problems later on due to the sugar content.

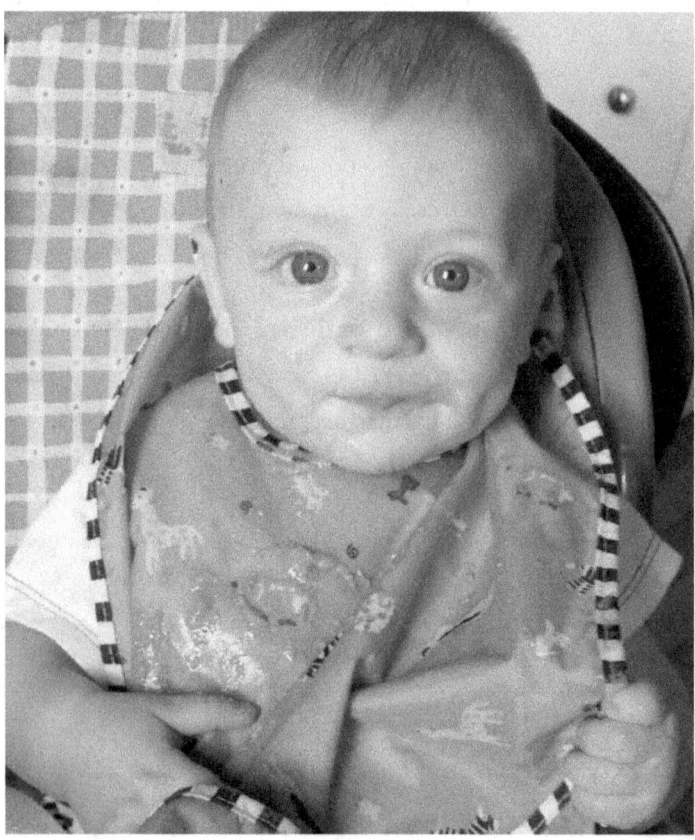

Let your baby try and feed himself. It will not be a pretty sight, but this is important to help your baby develop his motor skills and sense of independence.

# Your Baby's height and weight:

All parents are naturally concerned about their baby's development and whether his height and weight is normal. Parents will frequently eye other babies and compare them to their own, wondering whether their child is bigger or smaller than other kids the same age.

However, this is a matter that's out of your hands to a large degree, as weight and height are due to genetic factors, and not anything that you are doing right or wrong. Ethnic and nutritional factors can play a small role but basically, there's not much you can do to change the natural course of things.

## What are growth charts?

At each checkup, the pediatrician or nurse will measure your baby's height, weight, and head circumference, and record the findings in a chart normal ranges for babies of the same age and sex. This is to make sure that your baby is developing normally, and really, that's all you need to know, isn't it?

A growth chart shows the full range of growth for a specific age for male and female babies. For example, if your 3-month old girl is in the 50 percentile length range, that means she is exactly in the middle of girls who are taller or shorter, and perfectly normal.

These measurements are general guidelines to help your doctor assess your baby's growth and reassure you that your baby's development is progressing normally.

Bear in mind that your child is your child is an individual and not a classification within a certain group. He will grow and develop at his own pace. Just as in adults, there is a wide range of healthy shapes and sizes among children.

Some parents buy baby scales and download growth charts from online to weigh and measure their babies themselves. I really do not recommend this as it can become quite an obsession with some parents. Leave the growth monitoring to the pediatrician. As long as your baby is healthy and happy and seems to be growing at a normal rate, what's the need for additional fuss?

# Baby Talk - Language development in your child

The process by which a baby understands speech and communicates is called language development. You will see through your child that language development occurs at a very rapid pace from birth until the age of five. By the age of five, your child should be expressing himself very well indeed. It's very difficult for a child to develop language skills after the age of five.

The stages of language development dare universal among all humans and throughout all cultures. However, the pace at which a child reaches each stage or "milestone" varies greatly. This is why a child's language development is measured against general norms rather than compared with individual children.

Interestingly, language development if girls generally occurs a faster rate than boys. It seems like women were just born to love chatter and gossip!

Language development actually begins BEFORE BIRTH. In the third trimester, a fetus can actually hear sounds and speech coming from outside the mother's body and even learn to recognize Mommy's voice.

Infants are acutely attuned to the human voice and prefer it to other sounds, perhaps because it is their first introduction into the world until they can see. It's also been shown that babies are more attentive to higher-pitched female voices. As they grow older, they are fascinated as well by the human face, especially when it's talking. They begin to develop language skills through repetition and imitation.

# First Three Months

Crying will be your baby's primary means of communication for the first three months he will also display the following abilities:

- He will seem to recognize Mommy and Daddy's voice.

- Will begin to turn towards familiar sounds and voices.

- Quiets down or smiles when spoken to… awww!

- Begins to make gurgling sounds indicating contentment or pleasure.

- Will cry differently to express different needs — learn to listen for this.

- Will begin to make a variety of cooing vowel sounds like "ooh" and "ah" as well as grunt, chuckle and whimper.

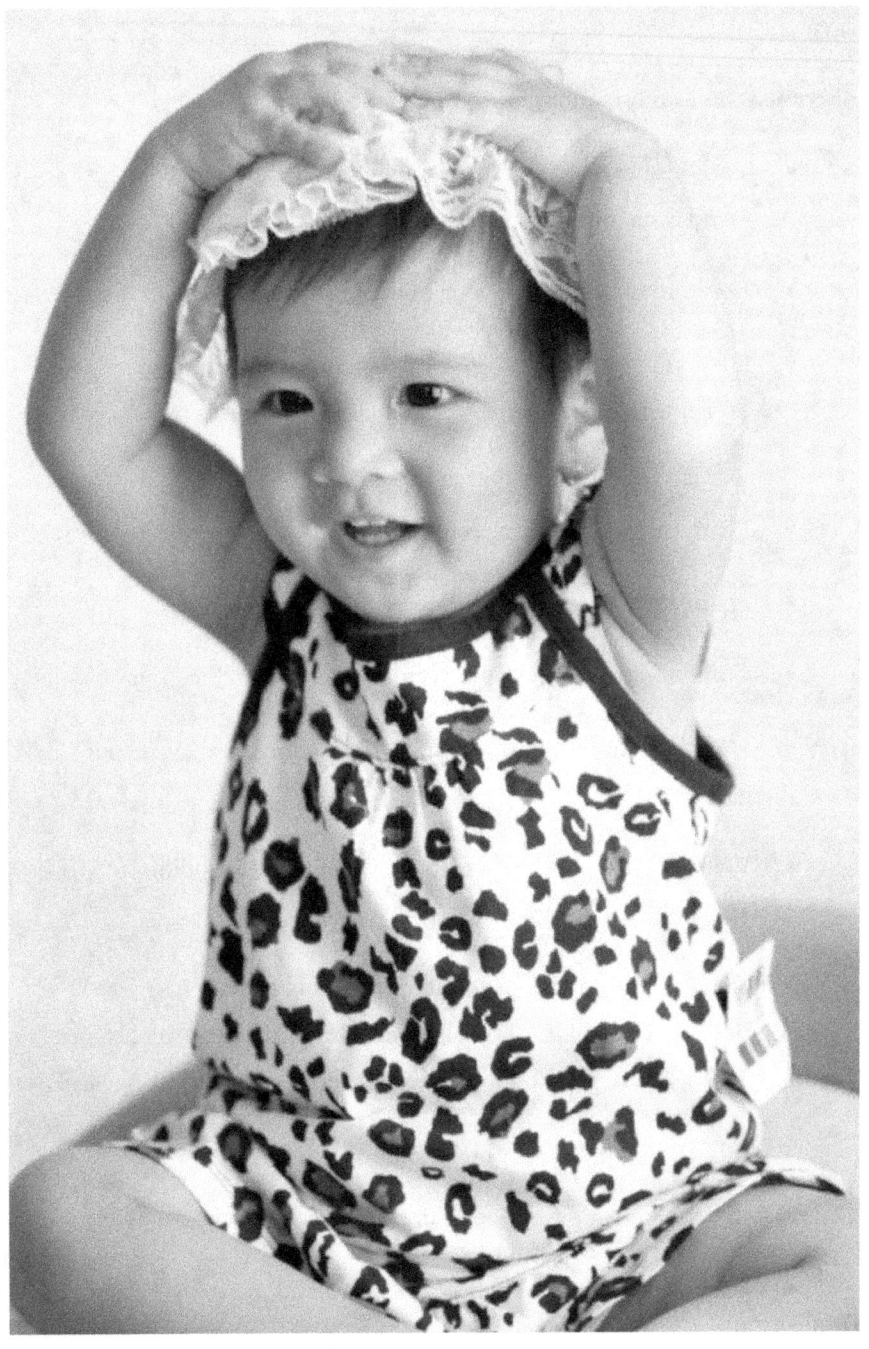

## Months three through six

Between three and six months your baby can do the following:

- Turn his head toward a speaker and smile if it's someone he knows – and even a stranger if he's a naturally friendly child!

- Respond to changes in your tone of voice and even cry if scolded.

- His sounds become more vocal including screeches to express excitement and pleasure – like when Daddy tosses him up in the air.

- Learns to vocalize displeasure with angry grunts and screeches.

- Sputter loudly and blow bubbles

- Communicate desires with gestures such as reaching out or kicking

- He will begin to mimic your voice inflections, and even your gestures

- Will add some new sounds to his vocabulary, including "p," "b," and "m".

Interesting fact - The sounds children make at this stage of language development are IDENTICAL in all babies throughout the world, even among those who are profoundly deaf. Talk about a universal language!

## Six through nine months

Between six and nine months your baby will start to do the following:

- Search for sources of sound , such as a CD player or TV.

- Listen intently to speech and other sounds and appear fascinated in conversation.

- Recognize "Daddy," "Mama," "bye-bye" and siblings' names even though he can't pronounce them yet.

- Will recognize and respond to his name.

- Respond appropriately to friendly and angry tones

- Express his moods with a larger variety of sounds and body language.

- Babble strings of random consonants and vowels sounds as if he's speaking an alien language.

- Begins to experiment with pitch, intonation, and volume.

- Discovers that he can use his tongue to change sounds.

- Begins to imitate your intonation.

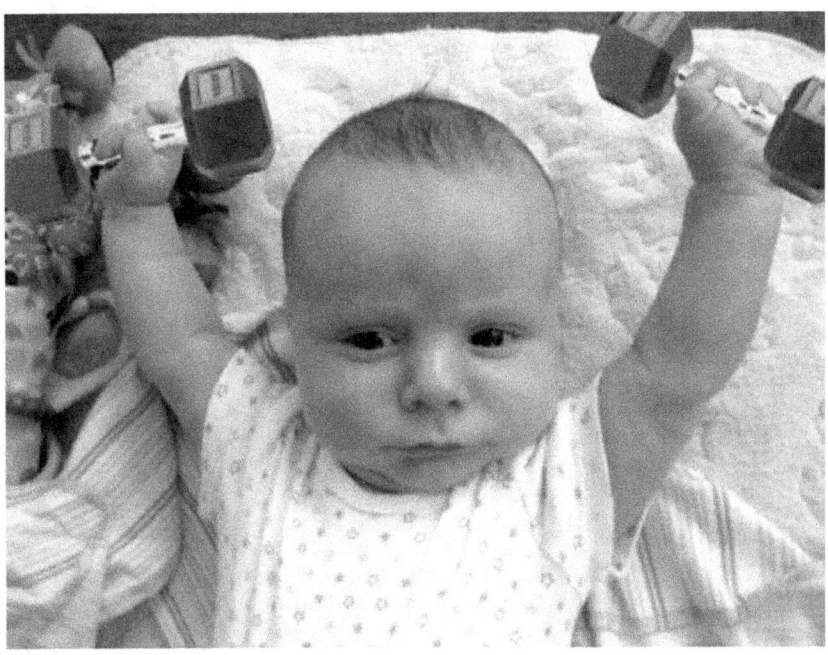

# Nine to twelve months

Between nine and 12 months babies may begin to do the following:

- Recognize words for familiar objects and names of family members

- Respond to simple requests: "Give grandma a kiss", "Open wide", etc.

- Understands "no."

- Understands simple gestures like "bye-bye" and "kiss"

- Associate the names of people with their voices.

- Speaks in full-fledged baby language with a large variety of sounds and inflections.

- Can say "Mama" and "Dada".

- Shout and screams in baby language.

- Tries to repeat your sounds.

## How to encourage language development

**Talk!** Studies have shown that children of talkative parents learn double the vocabulary as those of not to talkative parents.

Along these same lines, a study by The National Institute of Child Health and Human Development found that children in high-quality childcare environments also had larger vocabularies and more complex language skills than children in lower-quality environments.

Talking to your child and allowing him to respond with a smile, gurgle or even an angry scream will teach him the art of conversation.

Studies have shown that frequent language interactions with newborns increase their learning capacity.

**Talk in "Parantese"** – This is the high-pitched, singsong voice parents use when talking to babies. Also known as "Motherese", it has been shown to enhance language skills.

**Sing** simple songs and lullabies to your child and repeat them frequently.

**Read** to your baby as much as you can. Enunciate words clearly and point out pictures to him and make your reading sessions fun and interactive

**Use proper words** for objects rather than baby talk.

**Speak slowly** to your baby in short sentences, drawing-out vowels and stressing syllables .

**Use animated gestures t**o punctuate tour words

**Comment** to your baby on what's going on around your and point out sounds in the environment .

## Language Delay

A baby's delay in learning to talk is the most common childhood developmental issue and is caused by several factors both environmental and physical.

The good news is that 60 percent of language delays in children under age three simply resolve on their own and the child speaks normally.

Language delay can result from a variety of physical disorders, the most serious of which is mental retardation, a hearing impairment, cerebral palsy and autism.

If your child is late in learning to talk and displays any of the following symptoms, contact the pediatrician immediately:

- Cannot understand or speak words by 18 months.

- Avoiding eye contact

- Has difficulty learning or saying name of family members and common objects.

- Very short attention span.

- Poor articulation where you have difficulty understanding the child more than 50 percent of the time.

# Teething

A baby's first teeth are known as milk teeth, and actually develop but remain hidden while the child is growing in the womb.

Milk teeth start to push through the gums when the baby is about six months old and your baby begins the process of teething. Some babies start teething before they are four months old, and some after 12 months.

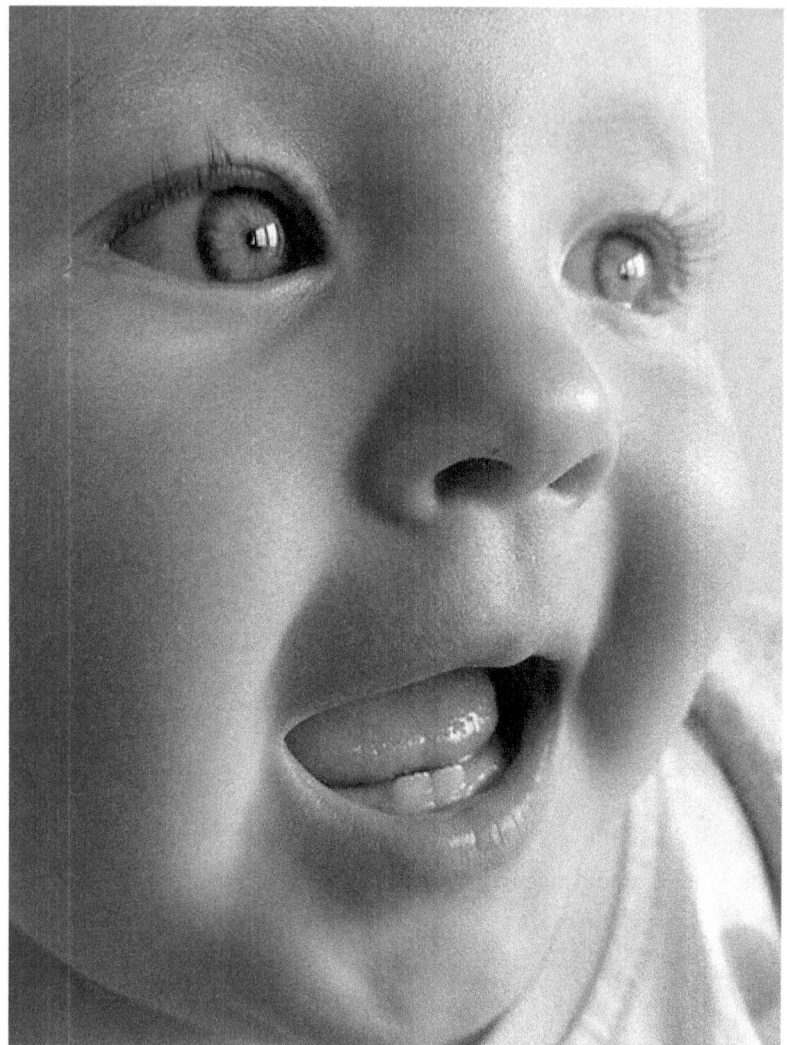

## Teething symptoms

- Some teeth grow in with no discomfort at all while other times your baby will feel quite a bit of discomfort and be very irritable. The most common symptoms are:

- Sore red gums where the tooth is coming through

- Flushed cheeks

- Excessive drooling

- The baby makes gnawing or chewing movements and puts his hands in his mouth.

- Mild diarrhea

- Mild fever

- Irritability and fretful crying

Other than giving your baby a teether to bite on, both of you just have to weather it out. If the symptoms seem severe or cause you concern, seek medical advice.

## The Teething stages

1. Bottom front teeth – these are the first to appear, at five to seven months

2. Top front teeth – Usually come through at around six to eight months

3. Top incisors on either side of the top front teeth, at around nine to 11 months

4. Bottom lateral incisors on either side of the bottom front teeth at around 10-12 months

5. Back teeth (molars) – at around 12-16 months

6. Canines (near the back of the mouth) – at around 16-20 months

7. Second molars – at around 20-30 months

Most toddlers will have all of their milk teeth by the time they are two and a half years old.

# Caring for your baby's teeth

Some parents wrongly believe the milk teeth are unimportant because they will eventually be replaced by permanent teeth. But milk teeth are crucial for your baby to learn to chew and talk properly. Take care of your baby's teeth as follows:

- Once all the milk teeth are in help your baby clean them with a baby toothbrush.

- Avoid cavities by not putting your baby to sleep with a of milk or juice.

- Actively keep an eye out for discoloration or pitting as this could mean cavities.

- Give your baby water after meals to wash down any food remnants on the teeth

- Arrange for your baby's first dental checkup when he reaches his first year.

# Understanding your baby's motor skills

Motor skills are actions in which your baby uses his muscles. They are divided into gross motor skills and fine motor skills.

Gross motor skills are the movements your baby makes with his arms, legs, or his entire body such as crawling, jumping and walking.

Fine motor skills are smaller actions your child makes such as picking things up with his fingers or wriggling his toes. But it's not just about fingers and toes, or even putting things in his mouth to feel them with his tongue.

Motor skills are very rudimentary in a newborn and begin with his head, such as face, mouth and lip movements and move downwards as he grows. Your baby will next learn to control the neck movements, then the shoulders, then the back and finally the legs. They gradually develop so that by the age of two, he can do some things for himself such as eating and walking on his own.

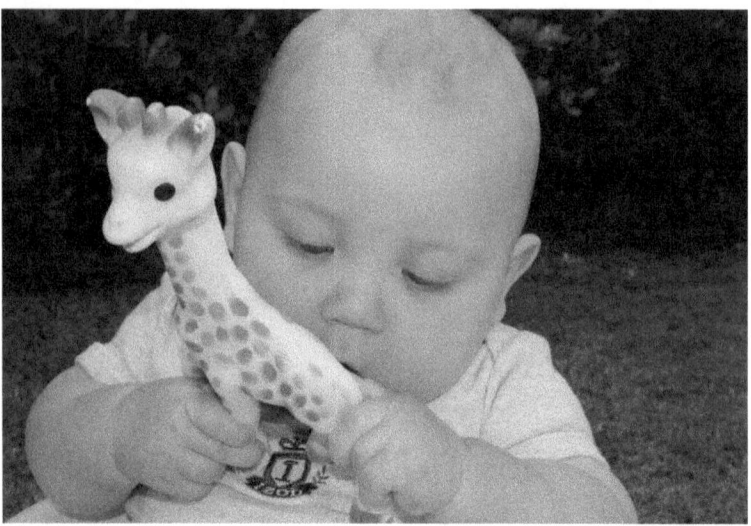

Encourage your baby to develop his motor skills by teaching him simple tasks such as holding a spoon or sipping from his cup.

Don't make things too difficult for him and move on to a new skill when he has learned the first, giving him time to discover and enjoys himself.

Changing your baby's position and activity frequently will help him enjoy discovering and developing his skills.

## What to expect?

For the first 3 months, your baby's muscles are undeveloped, and you must take great care to support his head and neck when nursing and carrying him.

By month 4, your baby has developed the muscle control needed to turn his head and follow objects.

From 4 to 12 months, your baby will gain the ability to balance, sit up, crawl, and eventually stand.

Your baby's fine motor skills also advance from clumsily dragging objects in the early months to accurately grasping objects and using his fingers to explore them.

## How to monitor and support motor skill development

Place your baby on his stomach in the early months while keeping a close watch to strengthen his neck and back muscles. Wave a colorful toy or make interesting sounds to get him to raise his head. Keep these sessions short, to no longer than a minute or two.

When your baby can sit up unsupported, play this challenging game: put his favorite toy just out of reach so that he has to balance to reach out and grab it.

Make an obstacle course. Place sofa cushions, pillows or lightweight cardboard boxes on the carpet and encourage your baby to navigate his way by crawling through them. Hiding behind an obstacle and playing peek-a-boo will make this a super-fun learning game for your little one.

Finger foods are a great way to encourage fine motor skill practice. Encourage your baby to pick up little crackers or bite-sized bits of fruit and veggies and lift them to his mouth. This game is not only good practice, it makes mealtimes an enjoyable experience. Remember, this should be when your baby is eating solid foods and with your pediatrician's approval.

At 4 to 7 months, help your baby practice by gently pulling him to a standing position. Your baby will start to understand how fun legs can be and start to bounce up and down while you support him. This is excellent practice for walking in the future.

**Bring out the blocks!** An enticing tower of blocks a few feet away just waiting to be demolished is the best encouragement for your baby to

Give your baby simple Jigsaw Puzzles with a few big pieces and peg-in-hole toys. Both are great for eye to hand coordination and your baby will find them mystifying and super fun.

Plastic "Doughnuts" is a fun classic that develops motor skills and helps your child learn about shapes, sizes and colors.

## How to monitor your baby's motor skills

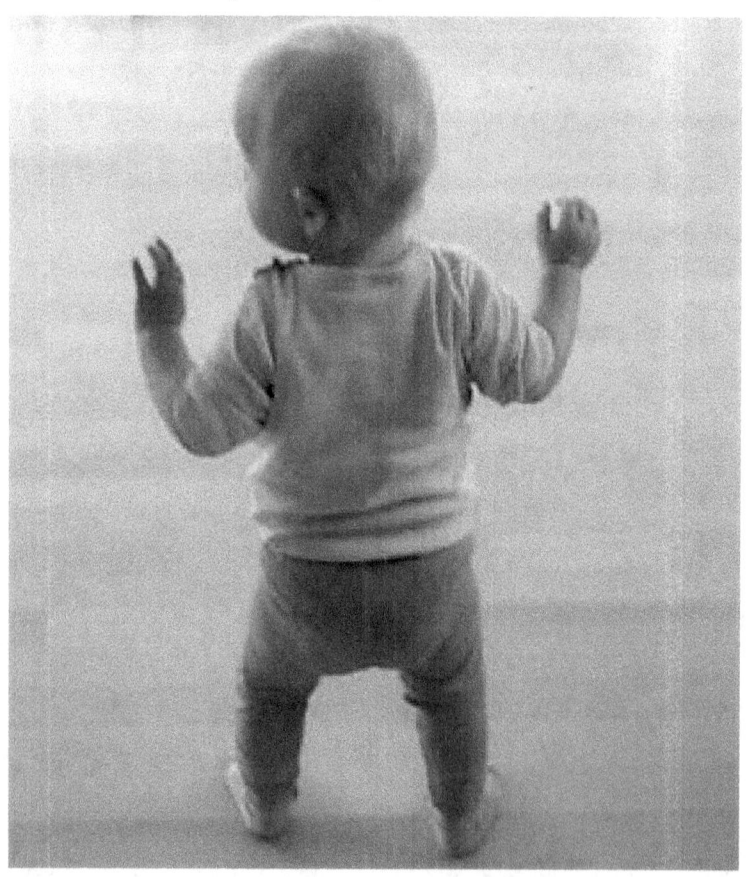

What will the crawling and walking process look like? Most babies exhibit the following developments between 8 and 13 months:

- First, your baby will be able to get on hands and knees and hold that position.

- Next, he will start to push back and forth and try to take his first movements forward.

- He will discover several new methods of moving around, such as swiveling and squirming on his stomach.

These experiments will continue for about a month, after which he will be able to crawl forwards. Don't freak out if your baby starts to crawl backwards instead of forward! This is common in some babies. As a matter of fact, babies have a lot of different crawling styles, from propelling themselves on their bottoms to crawling with arms and legs extended as if swimming!

Encourage your baby's newly-learned locomotion skills by playing fun games such as "crawl tag". Crawl slowly behind your baby saying "Mommy's gonna get you!" then turn and crawl away to let him turn and try to get you.

ELANE HOLLOWAY

# Immunizations

I probably don't need to tell you this but it is essential that your baby has the correct immunizations at the right time. Immunization has saved hundreds of thousands of children's lives since it was introduced, and we're truly blessed to be living in times when we are able to protect our children from many fatal diseases. Immunizations is a simple procedure where your baby is given a vaccine that makes him immune to serious, and sometimes fatal, diseases.

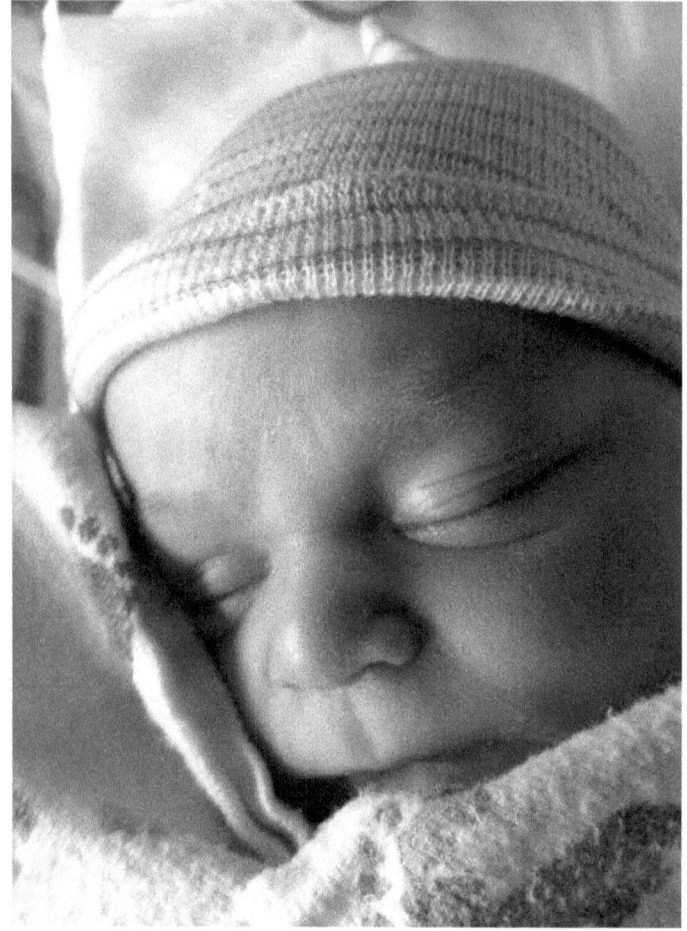

Babies are born with some degree of natural immunity that they acquire from their mothers while still in the womb. This immunity is furthers further strengthened through breastfeeding, as the mother's milk is rich in natural antibodies. However, this immunity wears off during the baby's first year, leaving him exposed to several childhood diseases that can be fatal or have serious complications. This is why vaccinating your child vital.

## Why are babies immunized?

When your child is immunized, say against smallpox, he is actually given a much weakened form of the smallpox virus. He will not get the disease itself because it's given in such a weak or form, but his body will produce antibodies to fight it. These antibodies remain in your baby's system so that if he is exposed to the real disease, he will be able to fight is off.

Your baby will be immunized against the most common infectious diseases routinely and your healthcare professional will give you a schedule for the required vaccines, which will protect against: Diphtheria, common flu, type B influenza, measles, mumps, meningitis C, polio, Rubella, tetanus, whooping cough.

Two other vaccines that protect against tuberculosis and hepatitis B are also offered to babies considered at high risk of catching them.

## Which vaccines do what?

To follow is a list of the most common vaccines and what they do.

### DTaP/IPV/Hib

This is a trio of vaccines that protect your baby against **Diphtheria,** a bacterial infection of the chest and throat which can lead to breathing difficulties and in severe cases, damage to the heart and nervous system, or even death.

### Tetanus

Or lockjaw, which can cause painful muscle spasms and stiffness, and can be fatal. The tetanus bacteria is found in soil and animal manure and enters the body through a cut or wound. It can also be contracted through animal bites.

### Polio

This virus attacks nerves in the brain and spinal cord and can cause paralysis. Thanks to the vaccine it has been completely eliminated in many countries today.

This vaccine is administered when your baby is:

Eight weeks

12 weeks

16 weeks

A preschool booster will also be given when your child is four or five.

*(Hib) Influenza type B*

A bacterial infection of the throat,   chest and ear that can lead to more serious breathing problems, meningitis and pneumonia.

*Whooping Cough*

A highly infectious disease

This is highly infectious and spreads through coughing and sneezing. The symptoms are similar to a cold at first but develop into severe coughing spasms with the distinctive "whoop". And become more severe. Babies and children are most at risk of developing complications such as pneumonia.

*Rotavirus vaccine Rotarix*

This vaccine protects against Rotavirus, A highly-infectious virus and the most common cause of gastroenteritis in babies. Rotavirus can lead to serious bowel infections and dehydration.

*Flu vaccine*

This vaccine protects against the common flu which can be actually endanger a child's life.

## MMR

This vaccine protects against three different attacks against your baby:

**Measles**: Although a common childhood disease, measles can have serious complications such as convulsions, bronchitis and ear infections and in rare cases, inflammation of the brain.

**Mumps:** A viral illness which causes swelling of the glands around the cheeks and neck. It can lead to meningitis, deafness and inflammation of the brain.

**Rubella:** This virus s is usually mild, causing a fever, a rash and swollen glands but can also have complications.

# Overall

Some of these vaccines can cause mild side effects such a slight fever, loss of appetite, rash or diarrhea. This is a normal reaction to the vaccine, and actually a good sigh – it means your child is building up immunity against the disease. Your doctor will inform you what you may expect.

With immunization, there is a very, very rare possibility that your child may develop an allergic reaction. These symptoms will appear within 10 minutes of having the injection and can include rash, swelling of the skin, lips or face, vomiting, or difficulty breathing. This is not to scare you off of vaccinating your child; the chances of this happening really are miniscule, only about one in a million.

You'll probably be asked to stay at the clinic for about 10 minutes after your child has had his vaccine, just to make sure he's fine. You can ask to stay a bit longer if you want to be extra sure your baby will be fine.

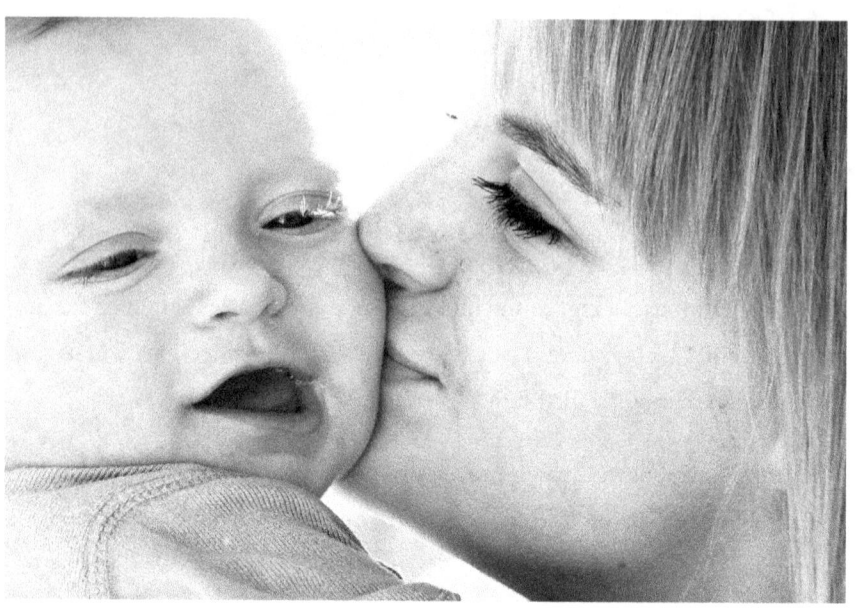

# Your baby's first cold

It's more than likely that your baby will catch a cold at some point during his first year if not several. Understandably, your baby's first cold will be a very anxious time for parents. Symptoms will include a cough, runny nose, sore throat and watery eyes, extreme irritability. These symptoms may also be accompanied by fever. A stuffy nose may make it difficult for your baby to breathe comfortably and will put him off eating. You can expect a cold to last anywhere from 2 to 10 days old, sometimes even longer.

If your baby is under three months old when he gets his cold you should contact your doctor. If your baby is over three months old you only need to contact your doctor if the fever gets too high, the cold lasts too long, or you suspect your baby may have an ear infection, if he has a persistent cough, or exhibits breathing problems.

# How to treat a cold

There are several things that you can do to ease your baby's discomfort and make him as comfortable as possible:

- Make sure your baby gets as much rest as possible

- Give him plenty of liquids especially if he has a fever.

- Elevate the baby's head with pillow under the crib mattress if he has a stuffy nose. Keep him comfortable by gently wiping his nose. Keep your baby comfortable by wiping his runny nose.

- Never give your baby aspirin for a cold.

- Let the cold sun its course. Lots of love, cuddling and patience are what's really required at this time. As worried as you may, your baby will ultimately get better.

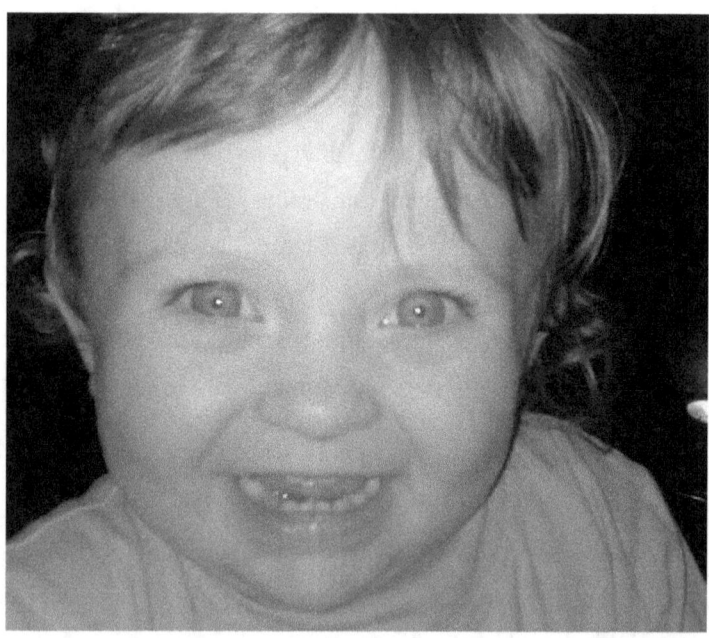

# Conclusion

A year from now you'll be amazed by how much your child has grown and changed, and you'll be proud of how much you've learned and accomplished as a parent.

No book, no expert can fully prepare you for the magical. Exciting and challenging journey of your baby's first year. Just remember that for every challenge or obstacle there will much laughter, much joy and tons of love. It will be one of the best experiences of your life, so keep your camera handy to record the precious – and fleeting – moments of your baby's first year.

Neither this book nor any other can possibly cover every up and down of your baby's first year, but I hope the information provided here helps you rise to the challenges and appreciate the wonderful new addition to your family.

**HAPPY PARENTING!**

# Other Books by this Author ...

## First Time Pregnant

### Go from Clueless to Confident during Your First Pregnancy

Expecting a baby and becoming a new mom is a very exciting time in your life. Unfortunately, it can also be very stressful –and at times down right frightening- if you do not know what to expect.

*If this is your first pregnancy, this is a must read.*

This book is designed for the first time mom to be as a basic guide to help you make the most of your pregnancy and prepare yourself for the changes you will go through and your eventual delivery.

Available on:

Amazon Kindle: http://www.amazon.com/dp/B00JYLN9HM

Amazon Paperback: http://www.amazon.com/dp/1499281919

Grab your copy today and be prepared during your pregnancy.

# ABOUT THE AUTHOR

Elane Holloway has spent her life with children. She has been a nanny, worked in day care centers, guided women through their pregnancies, assisted in countless deliveries as a Douala, and has raised her own children for all of their lives. She specializes in counseling women on raising children through their formative years. She was born and raised in Michigan and lives in the Detroit area with her husband, two children, and their cat, Motzart. Incidentally, she is also an avid Dr. Who fan.